First Due Trench Rescue

First Due Trench Rescue

JAMES B. GARGAN

Rescue Training Consultants

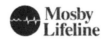

Mosby
Lifeline

An Affiliate of Elsevier

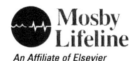

Publisher: David Dusthimer
Executive Editor: Claire Merrick
Editor: Rina Steinhauer
Assistant Editor: John Goucher
Project Manager: Chris Baumle
Senior Production Editor: Shannon Canty
Production Editor: Michelle R. Fitzgerald
Design Manager: Nancy McDonald
Designer: Ellen C. Dawson
Manufacturing Manager: Betty Richmond
Photographer: Les Lougheed

Second Edition
Copyright 1996 by Mosby, Inc.
A Mosby Lifeline An Affiliate of Elsevier

Mosby
11830 Westline Industrial Drive
St. Louis, MO 63146

Library of Congress Cataloging-in-Publication Data

Gargan, James B.
    First due: trench rescue / James B. Gargan.
        p.   cm.
    Second ed. of: Trench rescue. ©1982.
    Includes index.
    ISBN–13:978–0–8151–3431–2
    ISBN–10:0–8151–3431–2 (hardcover)
        1. Excavation—Safety measures.   2. Rescue work.   I. Gargan,
    James B., 1932–   Trench rescue.
    TA730.G325 1996
    624. 1′52′ 0289—dc20   95–36505

Permissions may be sought directly from Elsevier's Health Sciences Rights
Department in Philadelphia, PA, USA: phone: (+1) 215 239 3804, fax: (+1) 215 239 3805,
e-mail: healthpermissions@elsevier.com. You may also complete your request on-line
via the Elsevier homepage (http://www.elsevier.com), by selecting 'Customer Support'
and then 'Obtaining Permissions'.

ISBN–13:978–0–8151–3431–2
ISBN–10:0–8151–3431–2

10 9 8

Foreword

As you read this, thousands of people are working in deep, unshored trenches. Anywhere people erect buildings, build or improve roads, or even plow fields, trenches are dug to bury pipes, electrical lines, and other utilities necessary for our use and comfort. Working in these depths is dangerous business. Workers can be buried with dirt, trapped by heavy objects, or engulfed in water. Even more dangerous than working at these depths is rescuing a worker who has been trapped by something gone wrong. Specialized sheeting and shoring systems must be installed or fortified to ensure the rescuer's safety and to prevent further harm to the trapped worker.

Jim Gargan brings to us nearly a half century's experience in the emergency services combined with a parallel career in the construction industry. His vast array of experience makes Jim the nation's leading authority on construction related rescue operations, especially trench rescue. In this field, Jim has no peers. His pioneering approach to the subject was presented in *Trench Rescue*, the first edition of this book. Now titled *First Due Trench Rescue*, the second edition goes in further detail to present the methods to safely address more complex challenges.

By combining his easy to follow, direct style of writing with hundreds of detailed photographs and illustrations, Jim presents the proper methods to sheet and shore a trench in various states of failure. By using a hypothetical situation, the "Parkway Incident," Jim illustrates the procedures to properly handle a trench rescue effort from the first report of the incident to the final clean-up. This makes it easy to relate the principles and techniques to "real life." Each phase of a trench rescue is explained in detail.

I know of no other source as detailed or as useful as *First Due Trench Rescue*. I would never attempt to teach a course in trench rescue without first consulting this book. Use it as a safety guide, a reference source, a training outline, and an example of how any well disciplined rescue effort should be conducted.

Work safely;

Lt. Steve Kidd
Orange County (FL) Fire/Rescue
Squad 1

Co-author: *First Due* Video Series

Preface

Rather than attempting to "reinvent the wheel," when I decided it was time for the Second Edition of *Trench Rescue*, I have added new and revised text and pictures, while deleting that which has changed. The bulk of the First Edition has remained unchanged.

In this edition, we will add coverage on the use of walers, sheeting and shoring "T" trenches, "X" trenches, "L" trenches, shallow wells, and extensive coverage on a different method of supplemental sheeting and shoring.

Also covered will be a lightweight aluminum adjustable trench box that can be handled by the rescue crew, along with aluminum panels for supplemental sheeting.

At the rear of the book you will find a copy of "The Law" OSHA 1926.650, 651, and 652 for reference.

Acknowledgments

It is always pleasurable to acknowledge the people who helped in any way to make a project a success. Doubly so for a book because it means the work is finished!

I would like to start with the Gargan "family." Mosby Lifeline Executive Editor, Claire Merrick, who believed (twice). Lou Jordan, Emergency Training Associates, who kept the book alive with a second printing while I put together the Second Edition. Harvey D. Grant, my friend, brother and business associate of 33 years who passed away. All of the Rescue Training Consultants instructors who contributed in innumerable ways to our tried and tested methods of trench rescue/recovery: George Beasley, David Clark, Clyde Coble, Carl Craigle, John Czajkowski, Mike Donohue, Jim Fitch, David Heglund, Frank Hendron, Walter Idol, Ron Keane, Harry Kelly, Steve Kidd, Les Lougheed, Harry Metcalfe, Mike Moore, David Morgan, John Ostien, John Perry, Frank Puoci, Jr., Dick Rawls, Tony Talamonti, Joe Vattilana, Rocky Walker and John Whited. With a special thanks to Charles "Brother" Smith, Jr., who wrote the "Emergency Care" chapter, and Tom Carr for his work on "Crush Syndrome."

Other members of the "family" are Ray and Bruce Cole of Abbotsford, B.C., Canada, who have stuck with me over the years with the pneumatic shoring and a new design on a lightweight tench box.

To my wife, Barbara, and my secretary, Deanna "Dee" Belay, I can only say without your patience and dedication, the book would never have been finished. To my son, Rob, who started the Trench Rescue Course with me in the seventies, I bequeath the honor of any update or rewrite.

And finally to the newest member of the "family," John Goucher, my editor, many thanks for your help in putting it all together.

Walter Idol, EMT-P, Chief Flight Paramedic, U.T. Lifestar, University of Tennessee, Knoxville; Lieutenant Steven Kidd, Rescue I, Orange County Fire/Rescue (FL); and Lieutenant Thomas Carr, EMT-P, Montgomery County Department of Fire and Rescue Services (MD), were the reviewers and critics of the book. They shook me and slapped me back into the reality that you take nothing for granted and present the reader with the entire picture, nothing less. My sincere thanks for that.

The Knoxville Volunteer Rescue Squad (TN) did a fantastic job on the pictures, teaming with photographer, Les Lougheed. To be expected by the best!

A special thanks to others who supplied pictures: Deputy Chief David Hayes, Cobb County Fire Department (GA); "Doc" Holiday, Montgomery County Department of Fire and Rescue Services (MD); Fairfax County Fire/Rescue Department (VA); P.J. Richardson, Reeves Manufacturing, Frederick, MD; Bobby Kyle, International Safety Instruments Inc., Lawrenceville, GA; and David Dalrymple, Clinton Rescue Squad (NJ).

And finally, my appreciation to Dennis Hare, Developmental Editor, and Robin Keeran, Project Manager of the now successful "First Due Rescue Series," and their crew, for their help in setting up the filming sequence.

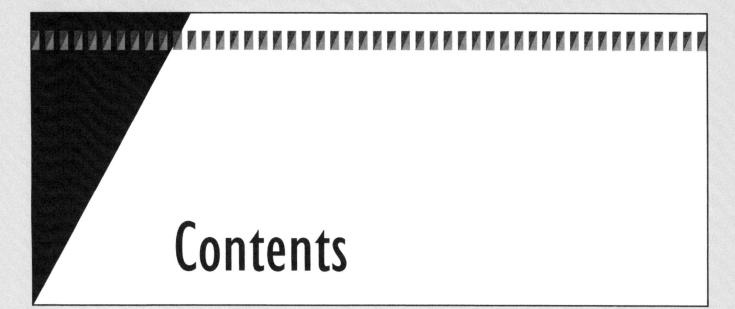

Contents

PHASE I   1

Preparation

PHASE II   25

Response

PHASE III   39

Assessment

PHASE IV   57

Hazard Control

PHASE X ▚ 205

Termination

APPENDICES ▚ 215

GLOSSARY ▚ 244

PHASE I

Preparation

KNOWLEDGE OBJECTIVES

The rescuer should be able to—

☑ Define relevant words and phrases
☑ Summarize activities of the preparation phase of a trench rescue operation
☑ State the OSHA requirement for making a trench safe
☑ List at least six trench accident situations in which a workman or workmen can be trapped
☑ List at least six conditions that are likely to bring about the collapse of a trench wall
☑ Describe three ways in which a contractor may make a trench safe
☑ Classify types of soil into three categories by observation
☑ List at least three mechanisms of entrapment other than dirt
☑ Relate the two ways in which a rescue squad can become prepared for a trench rescue operation
☑ Describe two types of sheeting that are available for a trench rescue operation
☑ Describe the form and purpose of uprights
☑ List and describe three types of shoring available for trench rescue operations
☑ List tools and appliances that will be useful in a trench rescue operation
☑ Assess an individual rescue unit's preparedness for a trench rescue effort

SKILL OBJECTIVES

The rescuer working individually or as part of a team should be able to—

☑ Prepare sheeting materials for use
☑ Prepare uprights for use
☑ Prepare shoring devices for use

WORDS AND PHRASES YOU MAY BE SEEING FOR THE FIRST TIME

Backfill. The refilling of a trench; or, as a noun, the material used to refill a trench.

Backhoe. An excavating machine that is equipped with an articulating boom and a bucket. May have crawler tracks or rubber tires.

Bedding. Sand or fine stone that is placed in the bottom of a trench as the foundation for a pipe.

Benching. Protecting against cave-ins by cutting the sides of the excavation to a step or a series of steps with vertical sides between levels.

Cave-in. The collapse of unsupported trench walls.

Check. A lengthwise separation of wood fibers, usually extending across the annular rings. Checks commonly result from stresses set up in wood during the seasoning process.

Compact soil. Soil that is hard and stable in appearance. Compact soil can be readily indented by the thumb but penetrated only with great difficulty.

Competent person. One who is capable of identifying existing and potential hazards in the surroundings or working conditions that are unsanitary, unsafe or dangerous to employers, and who has authorization to take prompt corrective measures. Required by OSHA on every excavation job.

Damage. With regard to lumber: injuries such as gouges, splits, and punctures.

Decay. The decomposition of wood substances as a result of fungi.

Disturbed soil. Ground that has been previously excavated.

Double-head nail. A nail that is provided with a flange close to the head. The flange prevents the nail from being driven all the way in. Removal is easy because the head remains exposed.

Driving home pipe. Connecting together pieces of slip-joint pipe.

Excavation. An opening in the ground that results from a digging effort.

Freestanding time. The period of time during which trench walls remain unsupported after excavation.

Kiln-dried (lumber). Lumber that is artificially dried in an ovenlike structure.

Knot. A hard, irregular lump formed at the point where a branch grows out of the trunk of a tree.

Laser blower. A motor-driven fan (usually 12 V) used by contractors to purge a pipe of stale air when a laser instrument is being used.

Mechanical strut. An adjustable support. When it is made up into a solid support, it resists forces exerted in the direction of its length.

Mudsills. Wales installed at the toe of a trench wall.

OSHA. The Occupational Safety and Health Administration, a division of the U. S. Department of Labor.

Pallets. Portable platforms of wood or metal used for the storage and movement of materials and packages.

Panels. Multilayered sheets of wood, usually 4 feet by 8 feet by various thicknesses, used to support the walls of a trench.

Pipe. A conduit for fluids, gases, and finely divided solid materials.

Pneumatic shoring. Trench shores or jacks with movable parts that are operated by the action of a compressed gas.

Right of way. A strip of land temporarily granted to a contractor so that he can perform his work.

Running soil. Loose, freely flowing soil such as sugar sand.

Safing. Making a portion of a trench safe by the installation of sheeting and shoring.

Saturated soil. Soil that contains an unusually high quantity of water. Easily identified because of seeping.

Scab. A short piece of lumber—generally cut from 2- by 4-inch stock—that is nailed to an upright to prevent the shifting of a shore.

Screw jack. A trench shore or jack with interchangeable threaded parts. The threading allows the jack to be lengthened or shortened.

Self-dumping valve. A spring-loaded valve that is part of a pneumatic shoring system. When the valve handle is depressed, the system is pressurized. When the valve handle is released, pressure is released.

Shake. A separation along the grain of lumber.

Shear. In this case, force-caused stress that results in the sliding of a section of trench wall from the main body of earth.

Sheeting. Generally speaking, wood planks and wood panels that support trench walls when held in place with shoring.

Shoring. The general term used for lengths of timber, screw jacks, pneumatic jacks, and other devices that can be used to hold sheeting against trench walls. Individual supports are called shores, crossbraces, and struts.

Skip-shoring. The procedure for supporting trench walls with uprights and shores at spaced intervals.

Sliding choker. A steel hook provided on a wire rope sling. The hook enables the sling to adjust for loads of various sizes and shapes.

Slope of grain. In lumber, the angle formed between the direction of the fibers and the long axis of the piece; usually expressed as a ratio of rise to run, for example, 1:20.

Slough-in. The collapse of a portion of trench wall in such a fashion that an overhang remains.

Soil typing. Determining properties of soil such as strength, in-place unit weight, compressibility, and permeability.

Solid sheeting. The procedure for supporting trench walls with sections of sheeting butted together. Also referred to as "closed sheeting."

Split. With regard to lumber, a separation of wood parallel to the fiber direction. Splits result from the tearing apart of wood cells.

Spoil pile. The heap of material excavated from a trench.

Spot-bracing. Another term for "skip-shoring."

Strongback. See *Uprights*.

Tight sheeting. Tongue-and-grooved timber planks.

Toe. The bottom of the trench wall.

Trench. A temporary excavation in which the length of the bottom exceeds the width of the bottom. The term "trench" is generally limited to excavations that are less than 15 feet wide at the bottom and less than 20 feet deep.

Trench box. A steel, fiberglass, or aluminum structure that is placed in a trench to protect workers from the collapse of the trench walls, and which can be moved along as work progresses.

Trench lip. The edge of a trench.

Uprights. Generally speaking, planks that are held in place against sections of sheeting with shores. Uprights add strength to the shoring system. They distribute forces exerted by trench walls and counterforces exerted by shores over wider areas of the sheeting.

Virgin soil. Ground that has never been excavated.

Wales. Braces that are placed horizontally against sheeting. Wales transmit loading from the sheeting to shores. Also called "walers" and "stringers."

Wall. The side of a trench from the lip to the floor. Also called the "face."

Wane. An edge or corner defect in lumber characterized by the presence of bark or the lack of wood.

Warp. A twist or curve in lumber that was originally straight.

Whip hose. In a pneumatic shoring system, the length of hose that carries air from the self-dumping valve to the quick-disconnect coupling.

Wire rope. An extremely strong rope made of strands of wire.

Wire rope sling. A lifting device that is made of wire rope. An eye is provided at both ends.

To function effectively, a community's fire department or emergency medical service rescue system must be prepared not only for the routine calls it frequently receives but also for emergencies of an unusual nature. A trench accident is a good example of an unusual and infrequent emergency situation.

Note that the term "system" is used instead of the more familiar term "squad". "Squad" denotes the physical and human resources that are generally associated with an emergency service unit: a vehicle, general and specific tools and appliances, quarters for housing the vehicle and its equipment, and a crew that comprises specially trained rescuers and officers. A rescue squad's equipment and expertise may not be adequate in unusual emergency situations, however. There may be a need for more specialized equipment and expertise.

There are two ways a rescue unit can prepare for situations that may tax its routine capabilities. It can be equipped with uncommon tools and appliances and staffed with persons who are expert in unusual rescue procedures. Or, it can gather and have immediately available for rescue activities a wide variety of equipment and human services that are collectively called "community resources." Whatever the case, with the addition of specialized equipment and technological expertise, a rescue squad becomes a rescue system.

Preparing a rescue system for trench rescue operations involves more than acquiring equipment. Dispatchers must be trained to elicit from callers specific information that will be useful to decision-making officers. Rescuers must be trained to use uncommon as well as ordinary tools in unfamiliar situations. Officers must be trained to lead rescuers while under pressures that may not be experienced in "everyday" incidents. And the community resources that may be required to manage the emergency must be recruited *before* the event, not after the call for help is received.

In this phase we will discuss ways in which a rescue unit can prepare for a trench rescue effort, either by becoming self-sufficient or by combining forces with community resources.

Understanding the Problem of Trench Accidents

There are all sorts of trenches dug for a wide variety of reasons. Some trenches are dug by a machine that resembles a Ferris wheel, creating an opening just wide enough to accommodate a conduit or a small-diameter pipe. Such trenches usually present little more than tripping hazards to workmen. On the other hand, excavations made for irrigation pipes may be as much as 30 feet in diameter. Although there are a number of possibilities for injury present at pipeline job sites—those generally associated with heavy equipment and heavy objects—unstable walls are not usually a problem because of the way in which the excavations are made.

Trenches dug by utility contractors for sanitary and storm sewers are more likely to threaten workers and pose problems for rescuers. Contrary to public opinion, such trenches are not always wide and deep. There have been unusual incidents of trench-wall collapse and spoil-pile slides in trenches 20 and even 30 feet deep. But statistics show that in almost 90 percent of the fatal trench accidents that have occurred in this country, workmen have died in excavations less than 20 feet deep. Significantly, the majority of fatal accidents have involved trenches less than 12 feet deep and 6 feet wide!

Illustrated on later pages are sheeting and shoring techniques that can be employed by trained and properly equipped rescuers in trenches as deep as 15 feet but no more. Accidents in trenches deeper than 15 feet create a need for special equipment, special techniques, and special expertise in trench rescue operations. The Occupational Safety and Health Administration (OSHA) requires that an engineer design trench stabilization systems for trenches deeper than 20 feet.

Federal law requires that all trenches deeper than 5 feet be made safe with either sheeting and shoring or a trench box, or by cutting back the side walls to the point at which dirt will not slide into the trench. Even though the penalty for failure to comply with these regulations is severe, there are still contractors who have no regard for safety and require their employees to work in dangerous environments. Their reasons for not bothering to make a trench safe are many and varied.

Some contractors argue that sheeting and shoring are simply unnecessary in shallow trenches, while others maintain that they can dig a trench, lay pipe, and backfill so quickly that there is no need for a safing operation. We might add to this group the "handyman" or "jack-of-all-trades" who thinks he knows enough to repair a broken pipe but never considers the safety aspects.

Other contractors attempt to rationalize their poor attitudes toward safety with the argument that the type of soil does not call for sheeting and shoring, that the earth simply can't shift! There is fallacy in such thinking.

Unfortunately, there are a few contractors who have no concern for safety. Characteristic of those individuals is the one who said, "It's cheaper for me to pay death benefits a couple of times a year than it is to go out and buy a whole bunch of expensive sheeting and shoring."

As long as there are contractors who either willingly or unwittingly allow unsafe work practices, there will be trench accidents. And as long as there are trench accidents, there will be the need for emergency service personnel to make trench rescues.

TYPES OF TRENCH ACCIDENTS

Consider what happens when there is a shift in the earth that surrounds an unsupported trench. Two workmen are joining pipe sections at the bottom of a trench that is 12 feet deep. The trench walls have not been supported in any way because the job foreman "thought they looked good." These men can be buried if—

- The lip of the trench caves in.
- The lips of both sides of the trench cave in.
- One wall sloughs in.
- Both walls slough in.
- An entire wall shears away and collapses.
- Both walls shear away and collapse.

Failure of unsupported trench walls is not the only cause of burial, however. Tons of dirt can be dumped on the workmen if the spoil pile slides into the trench. Such slides occur when the pile is placed too close to the trench lip or when the ground beneath the pile gives way. OSHA regulations specifically mandate a minimum of 2 feet between the trench wall and the spoil pile.

THE EFFECTS OF TRENCH ACCIDENTS

The consequences of a trench collapse or a spoil-pile slide are severe. Boulders and lengths of pipe dislodged during the movement of earth can cause injuries and deaths. But so can plain dirt, and not much of it!

In trench rescue training courses conducted by Rescue Training Consultants, rescuers are required to properly sheet and shore a trench and then reach and uncover a manikin that has been buried under 18 inches of dirt. As they remove the dirt, the rescuers are required to weigh each bucketful. In most cases the rescuers learn that the manikin is covered with 2500 to 3000 pounds of dirt, depending on the moisture content of the ground. Moreover, they find that between 750 and 1000 pounds of dirt are concentrated directly on the 4 square feet or so of chest or back surface (Figure 1-1).

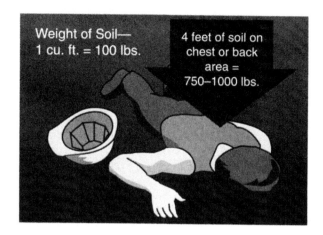

Figure I-I. Weight of dirt.

The conclusion? It is highly unlikely that a workman will survive such burial, even for a few minutes. He probably will suffocate, not only because of the reduction of available air but because of the severe compressing forces that will prohibit the chest and lung movements necessary for respiration. If this is not sufficient reason for contractors to make trenches safe for their workmen, it should be sufficient inspiration for emergency service personnel to properly sheet and shore a trench before jumping in and starting the recovery efforts.

SOME MISTAKEN NOTIONS ABOUT TRENCH ACCIDENTS

We have already considered the most common mistaken notion about trench accidents: that only wide and deep trenches collapse. Another misconception concerns the weather.

With very little imagination, you can shut your eyes and conjure up the movie-screen image of workmen laboring feverishly in the bottom of a huge trench, trying desperately to complete a pipeline before a downpour of rain causes a flood that will wash the job site away. Movie-screen image it is, for although rain may contribute to the collapse of unsupported trench walls, the fact is that most cave-ins occur during good weather.

One misconception about trench accidents has to do with the age of the workmen involved. Youth and inexperience often are cited as contributing factors when people are killed or injured in trench accidents. However, in a study of 64 accident reports filed by OSHA Compliance Officers, it was noted that 40 of the workmen either killed or injured were over 30 years of age, and 18 were over age 50. There is little apparent correlation between age (and perhaps experience) and job safety.

Another mistaken notion revolves around job-site safety practices. Contractors and rescuers sometimes think that once trench walls have been supported with sheeting and shoring, the trench is accident-proof. This is not so. While most accidents *do* occur in trenches that are not protected, cave-ins have resulted in deaths and injuries in trenches that have been sloped, in trenches protected by skip-shoring, and even in trenches secured with tight sheeting and shoring or with trench boxes.

CONDITIONS THAT CONTRIBUTE TO TRENCH ACCIDENTS

Utility contractors have identified conditions that are likely to contribute to the collapse of trench walls. Note that they are listed in descending order of occurrence, with disturbed soil being the condition most likely to bring about a wall failure.

- **Disturbed soil,** such as ground that has been previously excavated.
- **Intersecting trenches,** where large corners of earth can break away.
- **A narrow right of way,** in which case there is not sufficient room for the spoil pile to be placed a safe distance from the trench lip, nor is there room for heavy equipment to be maneuvered a safe distance from the trench lip.
- **Vibrations** caused by construction equipment, nearby traffic, or trains.
- **Increased seepage of subsurface water,** a condition that causes soil to become saturated and thus unstable.
- **Drying of exposed trench walls,** in which case the natural moisture that binds together soil particles is lost.
- **Inclined layers of soil dipping into the trench,** where layers of different types of soil can slide one upon the other and cause the trench walls to collapse.

The type of soil is also a factor that contributes to the collapse of trench walls. Look at the correlation between soil types and the number of wall failures in a study of 82 trench accidents.

Type of Soil	Number of Failures
Clay and/or mud	32
Sand	21
Wet dirt (probably silty clay)	10
Sand, gravel, and clay	8
Rock	7
Gravel	4
Sand and gravel	2

Note that clay is the soil type in more than one third of the incidents studied. This may seem un-

usual since clay generally conveys the image of a material with particles bound firmly together. Even though a clay wall may seem firm and unyielding, large chunks, and even whole sections, of wall can break away if the trench remains unsupported.

In short, there is no such thing as a "routine"or "standard" trench accident. The walls of an unprotected trench can collapse almost anytime regardless of the weather, the depth and width of the trench, the condition of the soil, and the safety record of the supervisor who deems the trench wall safe without support. Appreciating this fact, you are well on your way to being prepared for a trench rescue operation.

> **Remember**
> Even on the job site where safety is practiced as religiously as it is preached, a faulty judgment or a moment of inattention can contribute to a disaster.

SOLVING THE PROBLEM

Contractors can make trenches safe for pipe-laying and other activities with sheeting and shoring, by using trench boxes, and by cutting back the trench walls. As a rescuer, you will not have as many options. You may be able to sheet and shore trenches up to 15 feet deep if ground conditions are favorable. But when trenches are deeper than 15 feet, and when poor soil conditions preclude conventional sheeting and shoring at any depth, you will have to combine your unit's capabilities with those of community resources to complete a rescue.

To determine whether or not you can make a trench safe for rescue operations you must know the depth and width of the trench and the type of soil. Gauging the depth and width is a simple matter; determining the type of soil is not so easily accomplished.

CLASSIFYING TYPES OF SOIL

To the uninitiated, dirt is dirt; and, as far as types of dirt go, there is dry dirt and there is wet dirt! How fortunate we would be if categorizing types of soil were as simple as that. The fact of the matter is that there are at least fifteen different types of soil, and to determine a particular type requires testing for eighteen properties. Some tests must be done in a laboratory. Worse yet, soil typing is presently so inexact that two soil experts might classify the same soil sample differently. Appendix C (Appendix A to Subpart P, Soil Classification) will assist you in determining soil-sample classifications.

One technique for roughly classifying soils is to indent the surface of the soil with your thumb. Another is to squeeze a handful of soil to see if the particles cling together. However, these methods require that you lean over an unsupported trench lip to get a sample, which presents an unacceptable risk. It is therefore suggested that you classify the type of soil at a rescue site according to your observations of the trench wall and that you describe the soil with one of the following terms:

- **Compact.** Soil that appears compact or even hard, and thus stable.
- **Saturated.** Soil from which you can see water actually seeping.
- **Running.** Loose, freely flowing soil such as sugar sand.

Exactly how important are these observations to a trench rescue effort? Many contractors have a rule of thumb that they use when determining whether a trench can be made safe with sheeting and shoring. If the walls of the trench remain standing for 5 minutes after the excavation is complete (this period is known as "freestanding time"), it is likely that the sheeting and shoring can be installed without incident.

Therefore if you arrive on the scene and find that the trench walls opposite and/or adjacent to the caved-in area are intact and apparently compact, you can initiate efforts to support the unaffected walls. On the other hand, if the soil appears saturated, or if you see sand flowing freely from the trench walls, or if the walls have collapsed before your arrival, then you will have to work with the contractor or other emergency service personnel in another way to make the work area safe.

ACCIDENTS WITHOUT A CAVE-IN

When developing a course of action to deal with a trench accident, keep in mind that not all incidents involve the collapse of trench walls or the slide of a spoil pile. Workmen can become trapped at the bottom of a trench by lengths of pipe, boulders, and even wheeled or tracked vehicles that are driven so close to the trench lip that they topple in.

In any instance when there is an accident without a cave-in, the rescue problem will be compounded if the trench walls have not been made safe before the incident. Both sheeting and shoring and rigging operations may be important to the rescue effort.

PREPARING THE RESCUE SYSTEM

Remember that a rescue unit that is prepared for "everyday" emergencies (fires, vehicle accidents, etc.) can be prepared for an unusual incident such as

a trench accident in either of two ways. The rescue unit can become self-sufficient through the addition of special supplies and equipment, or it can join forces with community resources at the time of an emergency.

DEVELOPING A SELF-SUFFICIENT ORGANIZATION

A rescue unit is self-sufficient and ready for service only when it has a vehicle that can respond immediately with supplies, tools, and appliances needed for a rescue effort. Conventional rescue vehicles are not large enough, however, to carry some of the supplies and pieces of equipment that are suggested for trench rescue operations. Sheeting panels are 4 by 8 feet and they can be as long as 12 feet when they are prefabricated with uprights. Therefore if you wish to make your unit completely self-sufficient for trench-related emergencies, you must consider the addition of a special-purpose vehicle.

VEHICLES FOR TRENCH RESCUE

Wheeled vehicles that are either built specially or modified for trench rescue operations can be divided into two categories: self-propelled and towed.

Self-propelled units. The motorized trench rescue unit that is shown in Figure 1-2 is an excellent example of how an emergency service organization's requirement for a special-purpose vehicle can be met with ingenuity.

Cobb County Fire Department in Georgia uses a Ford 4 × 4 as their Trench Rescue Unit. From plans drawn by the training division, fire department shop personnel converted the truck into a unit that is completely self-contained, that is, one that carries sheeting and shoring and all of the supplies and equipment that might be needed during a trench res-

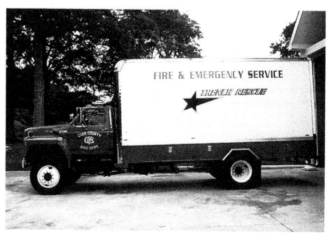

Figure 1-2. Cobb County (GA) truck.

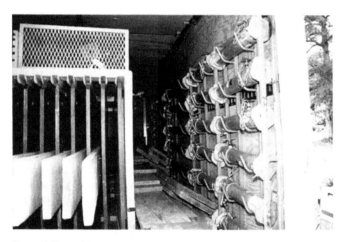

Figure 1-3. Cobb County (GA) truck.

cue effort. Note the manner in which the equipment is stored, particularly the way in which the heavy sheeting panels are contained (Figures 1-3 and 1-4). The Cobb County unit is housed in a central location and can respond immediately to any place in the service area.

Virtually any truck larger than a pickup can be converted to a rescue unit; the only real considera-

tion is body length. The body should be long enough to completely contain the 12-foot prefabricated panel and upright units that are so important to the rescue effort.

There are those who will argue that a self-propelled unit is not cost effective, that it will not be used enough to justify the acquisition and conversion expenses. This may be true if the unit is used for nothing but trench rescue calls. However, such a unit is versatile. It can be used in building-collapse situations, at vehicle accident sites where heavy vehicles must be stabilized, at train wrecks, or wherever special equipment may be needed to support heavy and unstable objects that pose a threat to victims and rescuers alike.

Trailers. Carrying trench rescue supplies and equipment in a trailer eliminates the need for a motorized unit. Knoxville Volunteer Rescue Squad in Tennessee uses a large open-top trailer, shown in Figure 1-5, to haul all the oversized special gear used in trench operations. Smaller equipment is transported in the truck.

The trailer shown in Figure 1-6 is used by Rescue Training Consultants for training. It is typical, however, of a trailer that might be constructed as a trench rescue unit. It is 17 feet long by 8 feet wide by 7 feet high. Note the manner in which the sheeting and shoring devices are racked (Figure 1-7). The trailer has a full complement of equipment and can be towed to an emergency scene by any vehicle that is provided with the appropriate trailer hitch and towing capacity.

A trench rescue trailer does not have to be specially constructed. Any of a number of commercially available trailers can be used as long as it is at least 17 feet long. It should have a heavy-duty towbar with a large-diameter ball, tandem axles, and a minimum carrying capacity of 6000 pounds. When pulling this amount of weight, all-wheel electric

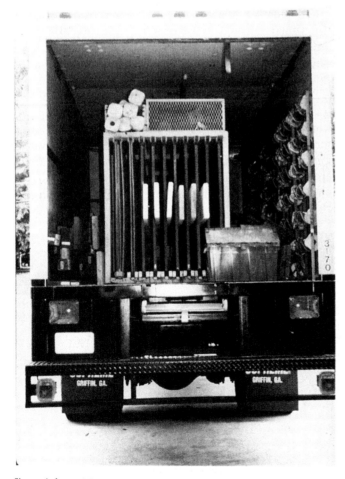

Figure 1-4. Cobb County (GA) truck.

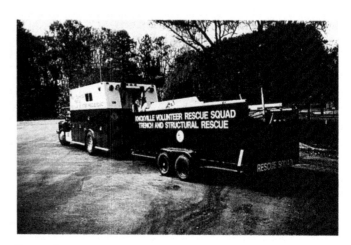

Figure 1-5. Knoxville (TN) rescue truck.

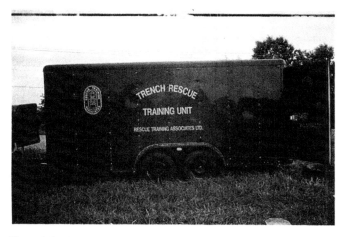

Figure 1-6. Rescue Training Consultants trailer.

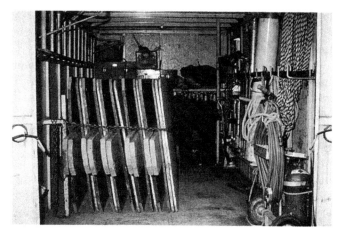

Figure 1-7. Rescue Training Consultants trailer.

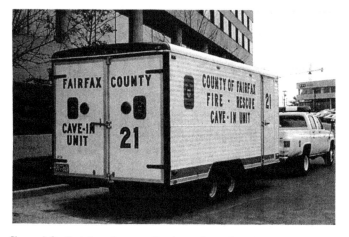

Figure 1-8. Fairfax County (VA) truck and trailer.

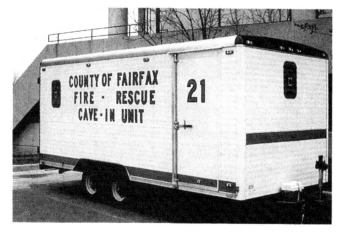

Figure 1-9. Fairfax County (VA) truck and trailer.

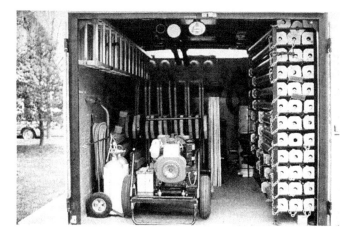

Figure 1-10. Fairfax County (VA) truck and trailer.

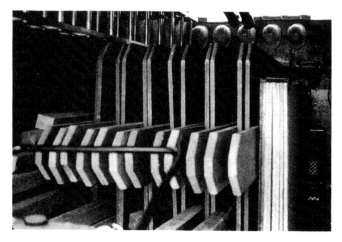

Figure 1-11. Fairfax County (VA) truck and trailer.

brakes with a hand trolley mounted on the dash or steering column are a must.

Fairfax County Fire/Rescue in Virginia uses specially designed trailers pulled by heavy-duty pickup trucks with crew cabs. The prefabricated sheeting is mounted on nylon roller bearings for easy accessibility. Enough pneumatic shoring to shore a burned-out building for investigative purposes is carried on each trailer, thus enhancing the versatility of the units (Figures 1-8 through 1-11).

A new concept called the "pod system" has been introduced to fire/rescue services by the Montgomery County Department of Fire and Rescue in Maryland. The pod system is nothing more than a Dempster-dumpster mounted on a conventional tractor. Yet the department has designed the box superbly, stowing efficiently everything needed for horizontal or vertical shoring. The advantage of this system is that multiple pods are available for different tasks (Figures 1-12 through 1-14). A support "tender" equipped with a crane, carrying heavy timbers for wales, and towing an air compressor accompanies the unit (Figure 1-15).

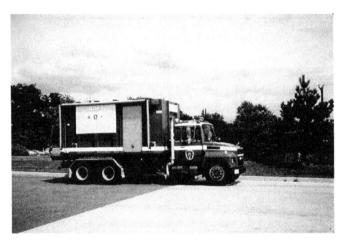

Figure 1-12. Montgomery County (MD) pod.

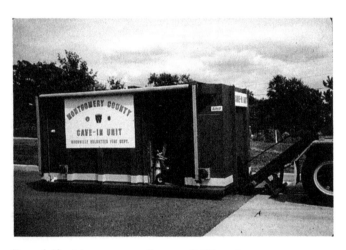

Figure 1-13. Montgomery County (MD) pod.

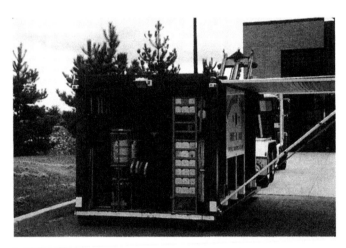

Figure 1-14. Montgomery County (MD) pod.

BECOMING SELF-SUFFICIENT WITHOUT A SPECIAL VEHICLE

Not every emergency service organization will be able to acquire a new truck or even a trailer for trench rescue operations, nor will every fire department and rescue squad be able to convert a vehicle for that purpose. Organizations can, however, become self-sufficient for operations at a trench accident by acquiring the special equipment that is not normally carried on the existing rescue vehicle and storing the equipment in quarters. When a call for a trench rescue is received, the equipment can be loaded onto a pickup truck and moved to the scene of the emergency without delay. In either case—whether self-sufficiency is gained through the addition of a special vehicle or through the acquisition and storage of special tools and appliances—requirements for supplies and equipment are the same.

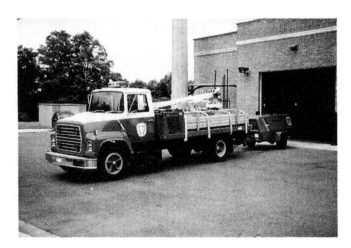

Figure 1-15. Montgomery County (MD) support vehicle.

EQUIPMENT FOR TRENCH RESCUE OPERATIONS

Diverse supplies and equipment are needed if a trench rescue operation is to be concluded quickly and successfully. Many of the tools and appliances listed here are of the hardware-store variety; many are already carried on rescue vehicles. But special items are required for stabilizing and supporting trench walls.

SPECIAL DEVICES REQUIRED FOR MAKING A TRENCH SAFE

Trench walls are held in place with a system of devices collectively called *sheeting and shoring*. Sheeting is placed against the trench walls and is held in place with shoring.

Sheeting. Sheeting must be relied upon to hold back tons of earth that can shift at any time. Yet rescuers often use materials that are woefully inadequate for the task.

Backboards are used as sheeting, as are wood pallets, sheets of $\frac{3}{8}$-inch and $\frac{1}{2}$-inch plywood, and even planks as small as two-by-fours.

True, these and similar items have been used successfully in past trench rescue operations, and they will undoubtedly be used successfully again. That there was no collapse of the trench walls is probably testimony to the fact that the earth did not shift during the rescue efforts. It is highly unlikely that makeshift devices such as those just mentioned could have withstood the forces of collapsing trench walls. The fact is, I have seen $\frac{3}{4}$-inch sheets of plywood folded like sheets of paper by the spoil pile cascading into the trench.

"Spot-bracing," or "skip-shoring," is a technique that is used by utility contractors to make trench walls safe when the soil is compact and apparently stable. Single uprights, generally 3-inch by 12-inch planks, are positioned at intervals throughout the trench and held in place with shoring devices (Figure 1-16).

Although skip-shoring may be acceptable for construction activities, solid sheeting for rescue operations—the side-by-side positioning of solid panels against the walls of both sides of the trench—is essential. Not only is solid sheeting stronger, it also has a beneficial psychological effect on the rescuers who must work in the trench. The completely covered walls have the appearance of strength and security.

Solid sheeting can be accomplished in the manner employed by utility contractors, that is, with 3-inch-thick planks, of random width, butted tightly together and held in place with wales and shoring (Figure 1-17). This is a rather difficult task for rescue personnel, however. The number of planks required

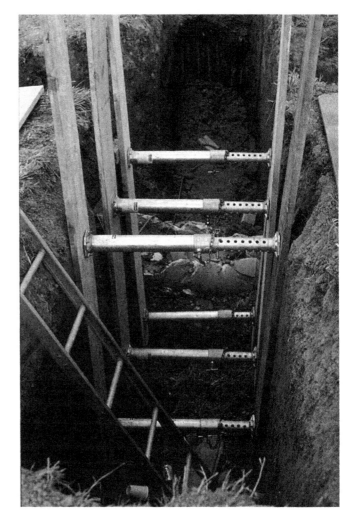

Figure 1-16. Skip-shoring.

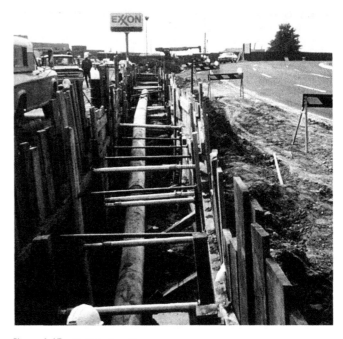

Figure 1-17. Solid sheeting.

for solid sheeting is not always immediately available. Moreover, positioning wales is a complex operation for someone not completely familiar with the technique. Solid sheeting with planks is a time-consuming operation, whereas sheeting with 4- by 8-foot panels can be accomplished quickly.

Shorform® is a type of commercially available panel that is recommended and well suited for solid sheeting operations. Shorform® panels are extremely strong compared to equal thicknesses of conventional plywood. This strength results from the lamination of layers of arctic white birch, one of the most durable hardwoods available. Shorform® panels are made in five thickness, from $\frac{5}{8}$- to $1\frac{1}{4}$ inches. One-inch panels are recommended for rescue operations.

If Shorform® is not accessible, plywood is available in a number of grades and thicknesses. Nothing less than the best-quality $1\frac{1}{4}$-inch exterior grade sheet should be used for a trench rescue operation. Two $\frac{3}{4}$-inch plywood panels can be made into a $1\frac{1}{2}$-inch panel if they are both screwed and glued together, rather than nailed, to avoid "slippage." These panels do get very heavy, however. Ropes must be used to hoist them.

Preparing sheeting for use. Shorform® and plywood panels should be prepared for use in the following manner:

- To minimize splintering, chamfer each corner by cutting away a small portion of the wood at a 45-degree angle.
- To facilitate handling with ropes, drill 1-inch holes in the corners of each panel 6 inches from the edges.
- Finally, seal the raw edges that result from the cutting and drilling operations with a water-base vinyl paint or thinned spar varnish.

The surfaces of Shorform® panels are coated with a phenolic resin at the factory, whereas plywood panels are left unfinished. Plywood panels should be similarly protected against water damage with a coating or two of high-visibility exterior-grade yellow paint.

Uprights. Sheeting should always be used in conjunction with strongbacks, more commonly known as uprights. When bolted to panels, these 2-inch by 12-inch by 12-foot planks give considerable strength to the 4- by 8-foot sheets. Forces and counterforces produced by the pressures of earth and the shoring devices are better distributed throughout the sheeting. Like panels, uprights should be specially prepared before use in a rescue effort (Figure 1-18).

First, chamfer the corners by cutting away a small portion of the wood at a 45-degree angle. This will minimize splitting. Then coat each upright with

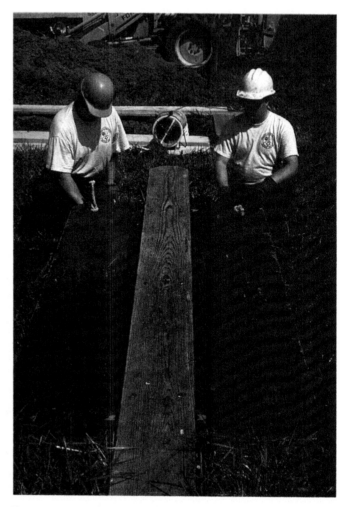

Figure 1-18. Panels and uprights.

a clear wood preservative. Do not paint uprights. Paint tends to hide dangerous checks and cracks.

The use of pressure-treated lumber for uprights, shores, or wales is fine. The only problem encountered is weight.

Uprights should be bolted to panels before they are lowered into the trench. It is the bolting that gives strength to the combinations of panels and planks, and the bolted-on planks serve as convenient handholds.

To prepare the panels and planks for assembly, mark the panels and uprights and drill $\frac{3}{8}$-inch holes according to the diagram shown as Figure 1-19. Take care in the layout; you will want all of the parts to be interchangeable. Some squads cut handholds along the edge of the panels with a router. Seal the raw edges of drill holes in plywood or Shorform® panels with paint or spar varnish.

It is difficult to suggest how many panels and uprights should be carried for a trench rescue operation. If you are going to operate a self-contained trench rescue unit, you will probably be able to carry eight or twelve panel and upright combina-

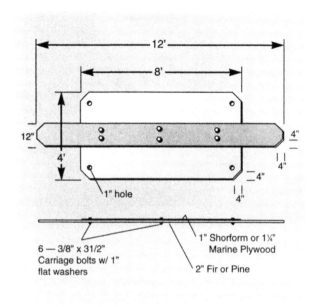

Figure 1-19. Panels and uprights.

tions. On the other hand, if you are going to store equipment for trench rescue operations, you may wish to keep only a minimum of panels and uprights on hand.

Six 4- by 8-foot panels will give you the means to solid sheet a 12-foot section of trench 12 feet deep or less. Eight panels will be needed for making safe a work area of 16 feet, and so on. To safely sheet and shore a 12-foot-long section of trench that is between 12 and 15 feet deep, you will need eight panels because of the different placement pattern required. If you have room either on your special-purpose vehicle or in the storage area, it would be wise to carry six, or preferably eight, prefabricated panel and upright combinations. This will eliminate the need for assembling panels and uprights on the rescue scene. If you decide against carrying prefabricated units, remember to have on hand a supply of $\frac{3}{8}$- by $3\frac{1}{2}$-inch carriage bolts and nuts and $\frac{3}{8}$- by 1-inch flat washers for assembling the planks to the panels.

Shoring. Never underestimate the importance of strong shoring. Shores must be able to withstand the forces generated by several tons of earth bearing on the sheeting they support. Shoring can be accomplished with timbers or with any of the mechanical and pneumatic devices that are especially designed for the task.

Timbers. Contractors have used timbers for shoring for as long as sheeting and shoring practices have been observed. Just as contractors use timbers to make a trench safe before pipe-laying or other activities, emergency service personnel can use timbers to make trenches safe for rescue operations. Use

of proper timbers is important, however.

When equipping a special rescue unit or storing timbers for shoring, be selective. Buy materials from a reputable, well-stocked lumber yard or building supply company, where sales-people are familiar with the characteristics and grades of lumber.

Although all sorts of lumber can be selected for shoring, No. 1 grade Douglas fir is a good choice. It is sufficiently strong and is easy to cut and nail. Douglas fir is normally found only on the West Coast. Southern pine is a good substitute on the East Coast. In many areas, only pressure-treated lumber is available. Other than the weight of the wood, there is no problem with using this material.

Select only kiln-dried lumber that has been stored inside, if possible, so that you can be reasonably sure that the moisture content is less than 20 percent. Lumber with this low moisture content can be stored indefinitely. If you cannot find graded lumber, examine that which is available for signs of damage that may cause the timbers to fail when they are supporting a load.

Inspect the timbers for—

- **Physical damage,** such as saw cuts or splintering that often results when piles of lumber are moved with a forklift.
- **Decay,** as evident from surface mold and staining.
- **Wane,** or a missing cross-section.
- **Warp,** which appears as a sharp bend or curve.
- **Defects,** including knots, checks, shakes, splits, and holes.
- **Insect damage,** or damage caused by termites and other boring insects.
- **Slope of the grain,** which should be straight-grained, that is, the slope should be no more than 1:20.

As with sheeting, it is difficult to say what length timbers should be carried or stored for shoring operations. Dimensions for shores are influenced by the depth and width of a trench. If you carry or store a stock of 4- by 4-inch, 6- by 6-inch, and 8- by 8-inch timbers, all 8 to 12 feet long, there will be few times when you will not be able to sheet and shore a trench with the materials at hand. See Figure 1-30 for a list of the sizes and amounts that should be stockpiled.

Screw jacks. Screw jacks are two-piece mechanical shoring devices that are used by many utility contractors. Like timbers, screw jacks can be used effectively by emergency service personnel during trench rescue operations.

Screw jacks are not always as strong as timbers. A 4- by 6-inch timber shore 5 feet long has twice the load-bearing capacity of a 5-foot length of $1\frac{1}{2}$-inch pipe that is fitted with the parts of a screw jack. **Thus you should not use pipe and screw jack shores in trenches that are more than 5 feet wide, unless you install two shores side by side.**

There are two sizes of screw jacks available. One has a $1\frac{11}{32}$-inch screw and is intended for use with $1\frac{1}{2}$-inch pipe. The other has a $1\frac{7}{8}$-inch screw and is intended for use with 2-inch pipe. If you elect to use screw jacks, be sure that the pipe is matched to the jack. If the smaller jack is used with 2-inch pipe, the jack can cock to one side when loaded, with disastrous results.

If you decide to purchase screw jacks for trench rescue operations, consider purchasing only the butt ends. By fitting both ends of a length of pipe with this combination of swivel base, screw, and long-handle nut, you will be able to adjust the length of the resulting shore over a greater distance than one made up in the usual manner. Also, use the larger jack and 2-inch pipe (Figure 1-20). A problem to consider with this arrangement is that you will be limited in the use of double butt ends in very narrow trenches, because the length of the screws will determine the minimum length of the shores.

Still another problem associated with screw jacks is that they can be turned out of the pipe when they are tightened against the uprights. You can eliminate this danger by welding a bead 4 inches from the screw end of the jack, as shown in Figure 1-21.

Since screw jacks must be used with lengths of pipe, and since the pipe lengths will vary according to the width of the trench, it will be necessary to carry or store a number of stock sections of 2-inch pipe from 5 to 10 feet long. And, of course, there will have to be a means of cutting the pipe. A good hacksaw and a number of high-speed hacksaw blades will suffice; however, you will be able to cut pipe faster if you have a pipe vise and stand and a

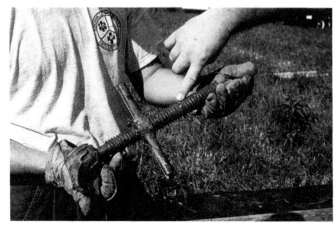

Figure 1-21. Weld bead.

long-handle pipe cutter with a reamer. The ultimate tool for cutting would be a rescue saw with a metal cutting disc. There are also chop saws made for this purpose.

Pneumatic shoring. Of all the devices available for shoring a trench, pneumatic shores are probably the most versatile and easy to install (Figure 1-22). Moreover, they can be used in virtually any situation: when the trench walls are vertical, when the trench walls are sloped, when there has been a collapse of a trench lip, when there has been a slough-in of a wall, or when there has been a spoil-pile slide. Pneumatic shoring is installed with pressure from a compressed gas supply.

The shore itself consists of a fixed sleeve, or barrel, that can be pressurized, and a movable piston. Shores are available in seven different lengths, from 18 to 144 inches (Figure 1-23). To allow for use in many different situations, pneumatic shores are available with fixed end plates (for use when trench walls are nearly vertical), and fixed or detachable swivel ends (for use when trench walls are sloped). One detachable swivel end attached to the bottom of

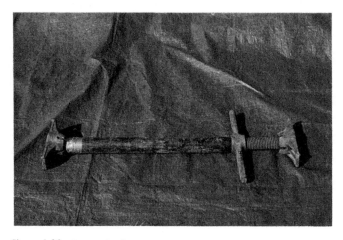

Figure 1-20. Screwjacks.

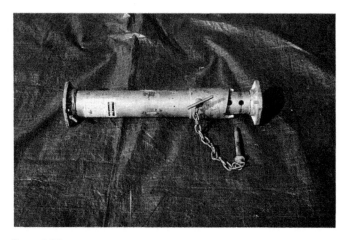

Figure 1-22. Pneumatic jacks.

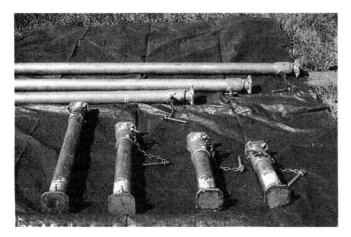

Figure 1-23. Pneumatic jacks.

the shore will give you, in most incidents, more versatility in placing the shore (Figure 1-24). Set screws are provided in the end plates. When these screws are extended, they bite into sheeting and help reduce slippage.

Pneumatic shores can be pressurized with com-

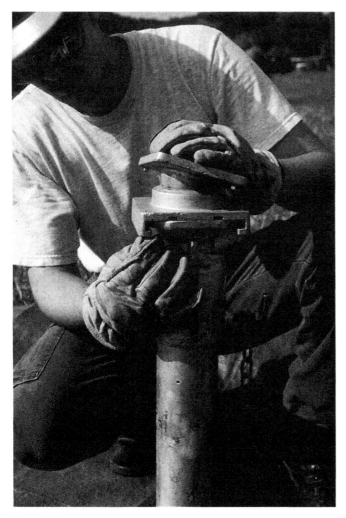

Figure 1-24. Swivel end.

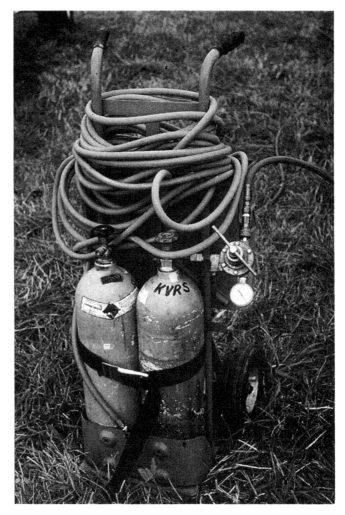

Figure 1-25. Carbon dioxide supply.

pressed air, nitrogen, or carbon dioxide (CO_2). A typical CO_2 supply system is shown in Figure 1-25, with the two cylinders secured in a welder's cart. A high-pressure manifold couples the cylinders to a regulator that can be adjusted to 350 psi output. The manifold reduces the gas flow from each cylinder and thus minimizes the possibility that the regulator will freeze during use. Fifty feet of hose connects the regulator to a self-dumping valve (Figure 1-26), and a 12-foot whip hose terminates in a quick-coupling device. The coupling mates with a nipple that is provided in the base of each shore. Pneumatic shores of the type shown are incredibly strong. Each can support a load of 32,000 pounds when made up into a mechanical strut.

Variable thrust developed in the shore assures that the unit is lodged firmly against the uprights. If the regulator is set at 100 psi, the thrust is 700 pounds. If the regulator is set at 350 psi, the thrust is 2450 pounds.

Although gas pressure is used to lengthen pneumatic shores, gas pressure does not hold the shores rigidly against sheeting materials. Pneumatic shores

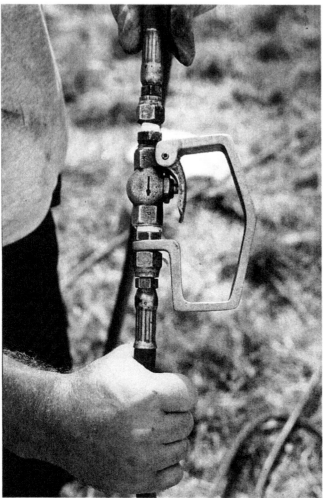

Figure 1-26. Self-dumping valve.

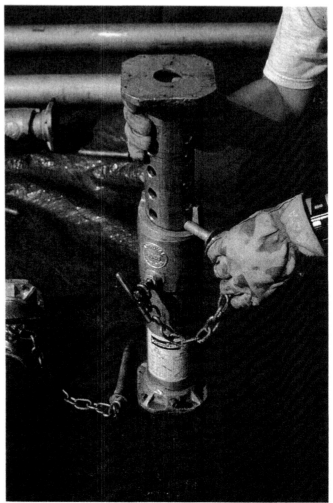

Figure 1-27. Pneumatic jack.

become mechanical struts as one rescuer operates the self-dumping valve while another rescuer holds the shore level between the two uprights. The piston portion of the shore moves outward and the unit lengthens until the end plates are lodged firmly against the uprights. The rescuer with the valve continues to pressurize the shore while the other rescuer inserts a steel pin through holes in the piston, rotates the collar until it is seated snugly against the pin, and locks the collar in place. The shore becomes a rigid mechanical strut that is no longer dependent on gas pressure for its strength (Figure 1-27).

The pistons of pneumatic shores normally cannot be blown from their barrels with gas pressure. Air release ports (bleed holes) are provided about three quarters of the way along the barrel. When the piston cup reaches these openings, gas is vented from the ports. This signals the rescuer to either select a longer shore or build up the space between the end plates and the uprights with planks, if the space does not exceed 6 inches. You can fill in the space with detachable swivel ends or by using additional 2- by 12-inch uprights.

In addition to strength and ease of operation, a real advantage of pneumatic shoring is that the units can be used in severe sand and mud conditions and even under water without fear of damage to the interior surfaces. If a shore is dropped with the pressurizing nipple face down, particles of dirt or sand can be dislodged by tapping, or they can be simply blown into the barrel! The flexible rubber piston cup will prevent the particles from working their way into the space between the piston and the barrel wall. When the rescue operation is over, clean the barrel by pulling the piston free, holding the barrel with the opening down, and shaking the dirt out. Other than cleaning the shores in this way from time to time, there is little to do in the way of maintenance. This type of shore lends itself quite well to structural collapse situations. It can be used vertically and can be placed by hand or pneumatically.

TOOLS AND APPLIANCES

Thus far we have examined the special sheeting and shoring devices that are recommended for trench rescue operations. Consider now the more ordinary

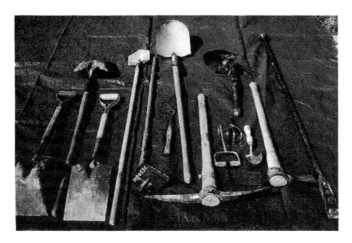

Figure 1-28. Shovels.

tools and appliances that you can use to bring a trench rescue effort to a speedy and safe conclusion (Figures 1-28 and 1-29).

Power tools. The only power tool that is really needed for a trench rescue operation is a saw. Recommended is a—

- 16-inch gasoline-powered chain saw with a case and extra chains.
- 16-inch electricity-powered chain saw with a case and extra chains.

A power saw should be included in the equipment inventory even though mechanical shoring devices are available. There may be a time when timbers or even tree sections will have to be used to add to the mechanical devices, and a good chain saw will assure quick and efficient cutting.

Although a chain saw can be used for a number of woodcutting operations, you may wish to carry a more conventional power saw for trimming planks

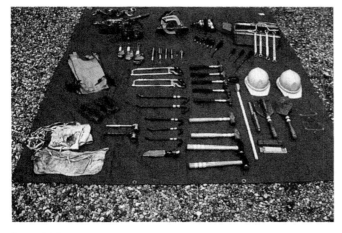

Figure 1-29. Hand tools.

and sheeting. A good tool to have is a heavy-duty circular saw with both conventional and carbide-tipped blades.

If you are going to obtain sheeting and shoring devices from community resources and fabricate combinations of sheeting and uprights on the rescue scene, you should have a heavy-duty reversible $\frac{1}{2}$-inch capacity electric drill and a set of first-quality high-speed drill bits or hole saws.

Electrically powered tools require a source of energy. Power can be obtained from a rescue unit generator or from a source on the rescue scene. If you are building a self-contained trench rescue unit and have the space, however, you should consider including a gasoline-powered generator or alternator, extension cords, a power distribution box, and whatever adapters are required for the different power tools. A ground fault interrupter (GFI) should be included on the generator.

Hand tools. There is nothing extraordinary on the list of hand tools suggested for trench rescue operations; everything can be obtained from a well-stocked hardware store. Even though they may be more expensive, buy only first-quality tools. They are less likely to fail when being used in a life-or-death situation.

A variety of striking tools should be included in the inventory, including—

- An 8-pound long-handle sledgehammer.
- Two 3-pound short-handle drilling or engineer's hammers.
- Four claw hammers, 22 ounce.

Dirt will have to be moved before and after a trench has been made safe. For that task you should carry—

- Two or more pointed shovels with long handles.
- Four or more entrenching tools (commonly known as folding camp shovels).
- Four 5-gallon plastic buckets with sturdy bail handles.

It may be necessary at times to develop leverage, as when a section of pipe or a boulder must be moved or nails pulled. Accordingly, you should have—

- Two 18-inch wrecking bars.
- Two 60-inch straight-shank pinch bars.

You should not guess at distances in the trench and around the rescue scene. For accurate measurements, especially when cutting timbers or pipe for shoring, carry—

- Two 6-foot folding carpenter's rules.

- Two 12-foot retracting steel tapes.
- Two 50-foot roll-up tapes.

Also suggested for trench rescue operations is a tool kit that includes a selection of screwdrivers, a hacksaw and spare blades, and a variety of pliers and wrenches.

SUPPORT EQUIPMENT AND SUPPLIES

A number of other items should be carried for facilitating trench rescue efforts.

Rope is always needed at a rescue scene. Since the ground around excavations is often wet, carry rope that will not be damaged by water. Include among your supplies—

- Twelve 35-foot lengths of $\frac{1}{2}$-inch nylon rope.
- Four 100-foot lengths of $\frac{3}{8}$-inch high-visibility yellow polypropylene rope (for crowd control and general purposes).

For protecting the trench from the elements during rescue operations, and for your equipment layout when the ground is muddy, carry two 12- by 16-foot vinyl-coated fabric tarpaulins.

Fuel must be carried for gasoline-powered tools and appliances. Include among the support equipment—

- One 5-gallon safety can for gasoline.
- One $2\frac{1}{2}$- or 3-gallon safety can for the gasoline and oil mixture that is required for two-cycle engines. You should also carry a supply of two-cycle motor oil so that the mixture can be made on the scene.

It may be necessary to secure shoring devices to sheeting materials or to build a ledge for timber shores and screw jacks. For those tasks, carry—

- One hundred 2- by 4- by 6-inch scabs.
- 50 pounds of 16-penny double-head duplex nails.

So that nails can be easily carried by rescuers, include six carpenter's aprons.

It may be necessary, too, to fill in voids between sheeting and shoring devices, or to change the thrust of a shore. For these tasks, carry fifty 4- by 12-inch tapered hardwood wedges.

Cutting timbers and fabricating sheeting and upright combinations will be easier when you have two saw horses or Workmate®-type devices.

You may have to remove boulders or lengths of pipe from a trench in order to remove a trapped workman. Even though the contractor's equipment may be immediately available, you should have two $\frac{1}{2}$-inch by 12-foot wire rope slings that have sliding chokers.

If you are equipping a dedicated trench rescue unit with a generator, then you might consider including four 1000-watt quartz floodlights with folding tripod stands.

Because of the problem of methane gas in trenches, you should carry a power-driven, high-velocity fan. Suggested is minimum 1000 cfm unit (such as a smoke ejector, a laser blower, or utility blower of the type used by utility companies) and an extension tube. Stay away from gasoline-powered fans if possible; if you must use a gasoline-powered fan, be aware of the flow of exhaust fumes.

Trench rescue can be a long-term, sweat-producing, energy-draining operation at any time of the year. For the benefit of your personnel, consider carrying—

- A 5-gallon water cooler with a cup dispenser.
- An assortment of quick-energy candy bars, high-protein foods, glucose drinks, or chewing gum.

And, of course, if you are going to use screw jacks you should carry—

- A pipe vise on a stand.
- A long-handle pipe cutter.
- An oil can with cutting oil.
- Ten 10-foot lengths of 2-inch pipe.
- A pipe reamer.

There are a number of other support items that might be carried, including battery-powered hand lights, a portable pump, and a few sections of hose. Determine your needs and supplement the inventory accordingly.

THE OTHER COMPONENTS OF THE RESCUE SYSTEM

Thus far we have examined the ways in which a rescue unit may be equipped for operations at the scene of a trench accident. Consider how the rest of a community's rescue system may be prepared for a trench rescue effort.

QUARTERS

There is not much to be said about a rescue unit's quarters with regard to trench rescue operation preparation. The following tips may be helpful to organizations that store equipment on their premises:

- Store panels and uprights prefabricated into sheeting assemblies, if possible. There will be no need for time-consuming assembly operations on the scene.
- Store sheeting materials vertically and on their edges. This will minimize the possibility of moisture collecting and damaging any panels

that are not adequately coated. If panels are not made up with uprights, provide small spacers to ensure air circulation.

- Store tools, nails, and other items that are likely to rust in a dry place. Protect tools with a light coat of oil.
- If you have boxes of supplies and equipment dedicated to trench rescue operations, mark the containers clearly so that they can be quickly identified at the time of an emergency.

THE RESCUE CREW

The finest special-purpose vehicle that is equipped with all of the suggested supplies, tools, and appliances will be of little value to a person trapped in a trench if there is no trained crew to carry out the rescue operation.

Squad members. Proper fire and rescue service staffing has become a serious problem. Budget cuts have reduced the numbers of career fire and rescue personnel in cities and towns all over the country. Work schedules, mobility, and declining memberships have combined to reduce the number of volunteers in these services. Thus it is absolutely necessary that personnel in all fire and rescue services be prepared to work under the restrictions imposed by limited manpower.

Two fire fighters can don breathing apparatus and enter a burning building to carry out search and rescue procedures. Similarly, two EMTs can work with basic hand tools to gain access to vehicle accident victims and even to disentangle them if other emergency service personnel are not available for rescue operations. In a trench rescue situation, however, it is highly unlikely that two or even three rescuers will be able to carry out the prescribed operations. There must be adequate personnel to manage a wide variety of hazards, to handle heavy sheeting and shoring devices, and to dig out the trapped workmen. At least six rescuers are needed, eight would be better, ten, better yet! This means that when an emergency service organization decides to upgrade its trench rescue capabilities, it must deal with the following personnel problems:

Availability. In the career service, a small rescue squad can be supplemented with personnel from engine and truck companies at the time of a trench emergency. Although the engine and truck personnel are not specifically trained for trench rescue operations, the rescue squad members are, and they can serve as working supervisors. If engine and truck company personnel are trained for trench rescue efforts as they are in Cobb County, Georgia, so

much the better. All personnel can then work together in the most efficient manner.

In the volunteer service, it is possible to train all of the active crew members in trench rescue procedures, but if there is a manpower shortage during daylight hours (when most trench accidents occur), there may be no more than one or two qualified persons available for the response. When a volunteer organization elects to upgrade its trench rescue capabilities, it should make every effort to cross-train personnel from adjacent communities.

Suitability. Besides availability, consideration must be given to suitability. It seems reasonable to say that not everyone is suited to undertake a trench rescue effort. A number of factors must be considered when selecting personnel for this unique rescue activity.

Physical strength is a must! Solid panels that are combined with uprights can weigh as much as 175 pounds. Teams of rescuers may have to carry several sheets for a considerable distance and then manhandle them into the trench. Moreover, rescuers will have to position shores, dig for buried workmen, move buckets of dirt, and remove victims from the trench. Each rescuer assigned to a cave-in unit should be able to lift and carry a minimum of 100 pounds.

Emotional stability should be considered. A trench rescue can be a highly traumatic situation for rescue personnel. Simply knowing that a person is lying under the dirt pile and may be unable to breathe may tax an individual to his emotional limits. Exhortations from workmen, police officers, bystanders, and even other emergency service personnel, along with the constant attention of the news media, will add to the emotional pressure felt by rescuers. Therefore people who are selected for trench rescue assignments should be able to remain cool in a crisis.

Resourcefulness is an important trait. Few, if any, trench rescue efforts are textbook operations during which the sheeting and shoring devices fit together like parts of a puzzle. There will be emergencies in which it will be crucial for rescuers to jury-rig materials swiftly and efficiently. For example, rescuers must be able to look at the slope of a trench and immediately decide how the angle can be overcome with wedges, pieces of wood, and the available shoring equipment.

Mechanical ability is desirable. A rescuer operating at the scene of a trench accident may have to cut planks and timbers, nail scabs to sheeting, assemble shoring devices, and perform a host of other hands-on operations. He should therefore have a working knowledge of the tools and appliances that are carried on the rescue unit.

A spirit of cooperation is essential, perhaps more so at the scene of a trench accident than at any other rescue scene. It may be only through the combined efforts of the rescue squad, other emergency service personnel, the contractor's laborers, utility company workers, heavy equipment operators, riggers, and EMS that a rescue effort can be successfully carried out. If the scene is filled with egotists and individualists, chaos will undoubtedly result.

Training. As for so many other emergency service operations, proficiency in trench rescue can be gained through hands-on training under the supervision of a qualified instructor. When an organization is self-sufficient for a trench rescue, its members can train with its inventory of equipment. When a unit must depend on community resources, personnel should be trained in all the techniques of sheeting and shoring so that they will be able to work with whatever materials are provided.

Officers. Rescue officers who will be in charge of a trench rescue effort must have all of the traits prescribed for crew members. They should also be trained in staff and command procedures because rescues are often long-term operations that involve many community resource organizations. At the very least, rescue officers should be able to set up and operate a command post.

WHEN YOU CANNOT BE A SELF-SUFFICIENT UNIT

Thus far discussion has centered on the preparation of a dedicated trench rescue unit or the storage of specialized items in quarters. What happens when it is economically or otherwise impossible to build a unit or to store special equipment? Does this mean that a fire department or rescue squad cannot operate effectively at the scene of an accident? Not at all!

OBTAINING SUPPLIES AND EQUIPMENT FROM COMMUNITY RESOURCE ORGANIZATIONS

Many of the supplies and all of the tools and appliances that are suggested for trench rescue can be carried on a conventional rescue vehicle. Items like bars, hammers, hand tools, salvage covers, and even power tools already may be included in the inventory of a rescue unit or a truck company. You need to add only the sheeting a shoring devices.

An emergency service unit that is serious about improving its trench rescue capabilities can assure the availability of sheeting and shoring materials without building a special-purpose unit or allocating valuable space in quarters for seldom-used supplies. It can locate the items within a wealth of community resources and make arrangements to acquire them at the time of an emergency.

Timbers can be obtained from—

- Lumber yards.
- Building supply houses.

Conventional sheeting and shoring devices can be obtained from—

- Sewer contractors.
- Building contractors.
- Mechanical contractors.
- Electrical contractors.
- Pipeline contractors.
- Highway contractors.
- Concrete contractors.
- Highway departments (state, county, city).
- Municipal and private water companies.
- Municipal street and sewer departments.
- Municipal and private electric and gas companies.

Scaffolding and scaffolding planks, concrete forms, and other items that can be used for makeshift sheeting and shoring can be obtained from—

- Roofing contractors.
- Park departments.
- General contractors.
- Plumbing contractors.
- Steel erectors.
- Painting contractors.
- Industrial plants.
- Quarry and mine operators.
- Refineries.
- Equipment rental houses.
- Cemeteries.

Once you have located the supplies and equipment that will make your trench rescue system complete, make a list that includes each item, its source, addresses, telephone numbers, hours of operation, and names of persons who can be called after hours. More than that, make firm arrangements with officials of the source organizations to acquire the items you need at the time of an emergency, and make arrangements with more than one place so that you can be sure of getting the items you need without having to call around town. When your source list is complete, give a copy to the emergency dispatching center. When there is a trench accident, the dispatcher will be able to initiate the equipment acquisition procedure without delay.

Remember
There is no fault in not having in-house capabilities for unusual incidents like trench cave-ins. You are at fault if you have not made arrangements for acquiring special equipment from community resources before the emergency.

When a rescue squad is developed into a functional rescue system that is staffed and trained, and either has or can obtain necessary supplies and equipment, it is ready for a trench rescue operation.

THE PARKWAY INCIDENT—
PREPARATION

Many authors create hypothetical situations to illustrate the rationale for doing certain things in certain ways. Authors of fire training manuals usually use words and pictures to develop in their readers' minds a situation during which certain firefighting techniques might be employed.

We will create a hypothetical situation, not only making one or two teaching points but keeping the situation alive throughout the book. Together we will see how a trench rescue effort can be brought to a successful conclusion by the combined efforts of rescuers and community resource personnel. And to minimize the impersonality that sometimes characterizes training manuals, let's say that you, the reader, are the rescue officer and that you and the author are discussing trench rescue techniques.

You are the rescue officer attached to the Meadowbrook Station of the Center County Fire Department. Yours is a quickly developing suburban area, with not only a great deal of housing under construction but several office building campuses and two rather large industrial parks.

The time is 4:00 p.m. It is a Wednesday afternoon. The temperature is about 80 degrees and the humidity is high. It has not rained for some time. Employees of the Edwards Construction Company are installing an 8-inch sanitary sewer line down the middle of an as-yet-unnamed street in the new Parkway Industrial Complex. A crawler-type backhoe is digging a 4-foot-wide trench about 12 feet deep in the somewhat sandy soil. Frank, the backhoe operator, is in a bit of a hurry, so he isn't being too careful about where he piles the spoil. It's getting close to quitting time. If someone were watching closely, he would be fascinated by the little rivulets of sand and stones sliding down the side of the pile and into the trench.

George and Henry are in the trench driving home the lengths of pipe. Since it is hot and humid, they are working without shirts and they are not wearing hard hats. What do they need hard hats for? There hasn't been a report of the sky falling since Chicken Little, and that's all there is over their heads—sky!

Pop Edwards has been in the construction business for more years than he cares to admit, and in those 30-plus years his people have never been involved in a trench accident. So Pop scoffs at the idea of using valuable time to install sheeting and shoring that will have to be removed after only a few hours. Because safety inspectors have visited another part of the industrial park only a few days earlier, he thinks they are probably on the other side of the county by now. Thus at 4:00 p.m. on a Wednesday afternoon the components for a disaster are assembled: dry, sandy soil; an excavation 4 feet wide by 12 feet deep; a spoil pile too close to the trench edge; an equipment operator in a hurry; hot, tired, unprotected workmen; and a "short-cut" boss.

At 4:01 the disaster is about to be triggered by the arrival on the construction site of an eighteen-wheeler loaded with 25 tons of crusher-run stone that will be used as bedding for the pipe. Pop Edwards looks up from his plans, points to where he wants the load dumped, and the driver backs his rig in that direction. George and Henry can feel the dry earth shake as the semi backs over the hard, uneven ground. Henry is about to laugh and comment that the truck would not have been able to get to the industrial park, let alone the job site, just a couple of months ago when the site was a sea of mud because of the spring rains. But the laugh catches in Henry's throat and then turns to a scream when he looks up and sees the spoil pile sliding toward him, having been set in motion by the vibrations caused by the truck.

In an instant, Henry is flung backwards over the 8-inch pipe, his arms outstretched as if to hold back the moving spoil. He probably feels a momentary white-hot pain as his spine snaps, followed by a numbness. But whatever sensations Henry feels he will not feel for long, because there in the open trench, covered by dirt and unable to move or even cry for help, Henry will suffocate.

George is more fortunate. He sees the spoil pile coming and, in a reflex action, attempts to jump over the fast-moving earth. He doesn't jump high enough soon enough, however, and he is pinned to the wall of the trench with dirt that reaches his chest. The pressure of the dirt makes breathing difficult, but, difficult or not, he is breathing. The scene is set. You are about to respond to your first trench rescue operation.

Remember

You are the rescue officer. You are going to respond to the Parkway Industrial Complex with exactly the units that would respond from your actual fire department or rescue squad. The only differences are that your units will be responding from the Meadowbrook Station and your radio designation is "Rescue 63."

How well are you prepared for a trench rescue operation? Take a moment and assess the state of your unit's readiness for this type of accident on the following form (Figure 1-30). Listed are all of the items of equipment that were suggested earlier in this chapter.

When you are finished with the form, you should be able to say "Yes, my unit is equipped for a trench rescue," or "No, my unit is not equipped for a trench rescue. I will have to rely on community resources for the supplies and equipment that I do not have."

1	Self-propelled trench rescue unit	☐
1	Trailer trench rescue unit	☐
1	Pickup truck	☐
10	Shorform® panels 1″ x 4′ x 8′	☐
10	Plywood panels 1¼″ x 4′ x 8′	☐
20	Uprights 2″ x 12″ x 12′	☐
6	Plywood ground pads ⅜″ x 4′ x 8′	☐
90	Carriage bolts ⅜″ x 3½″	☐
90	Nuts ⅜″	☐
90	Flat washers ⅜″ x 1″	☐
10	Timbers 4″ x 4″ x 8′	☐
10	Timbers 6″ x 6″ x 12′	☐
6	Timbers 8″ x 8″ x 12′	☐
12	Screw jack sets - 2″	☐
10	Lengths of pipe - 2″	☐
1	Pipe stand w/cutter & oil	☐
	Pneumatic shoring w/pressurizing kit	☐
1	Gasoline powered chain saw with extra chain and chain saw case	☐
1	Electric-powered chain saw with extra chain and chain saw case	☐
1	Atmospheric monitor	☐
1	Rescue saw w/carbide tip blade	☐
2	Dry diamond blades	☐
6	Steel disc blades	☐
1	H.D. Circular saw w/conventional blade	☐
1	Carbide tip blade	☐
1	H.D. ½″ reversible drill	☐
1	Set of drill bits	☐
1	Set of hole saws	☐
2	Sledge hammer - 8#	☐
2	Short-handle sledge hammers - 3#	☐
4	Claw hammers - 22 oz.	☐
2	Long-handle pointed shovels	☐
4	Entrenching tools	☐
4	(5) Gallon plastic buckets	☐
2	Wrecking bars - 18″	☐
2	Pinch bars - 60″	☐
1	Digging bar - 60″	☐
2	Folding rules - 6′	☐
2	Retracting steel tapes - 12′	☐
2	Roll-up tapes - 50′	☐
1	Tool kit	☐
12	Nylon rope ½″ x 35′	☐
4	Polypropylene rope ⅜″ x 100′	☐
2	Vinyl tarpaulins 12′ x 16′	☐
1	Water cooler - 5 gallon	☐
1	Gasoline safety can - 5 gallon	☐
1	Gasoline/oil mix safety can - 2½ gallon	☐
100	Scabs - 2″ x 4″ x 6″	☐
50	lb. - Duplex nails - 16pp	☐
6	Carpenters aprons	☐
50	Tapered hardwood wedges 4″ x 12″	☐
2	Saw horses or Workmates®	☐
2	Wire rope slings w/sliding chokers ½″ x 12′	☐
3	Portable generators 3500w min	☐
3	Distribution boxes	☐
4	Portable floodlights 1000w min	☐
4	Quartz floodlights w/tripod folding stands	☐
1	Smoke ejector or utility blower w/extension tube	☐
4	Battery powered handlites	☐
1	Electric submersible pump - 1½″	☐
2	Discharge hose - 50′	☐
1	Trash pump - 3″	☐
2	Suction hose - 10′	☐
1	Lineman's clamp stick	☐
1	Lineman's hot stick	☐
2	Lineman's gloves	☐
1	Synthetic fiber weighted throwing line - 50′	☐
12	Traffic cones	☐
4	Traffic flags	☐
50	Flares	☐
2	Wall ladders - 16′	☐
2	Extension ladders - 24′	☐
3	Self-contained breathing apparatus (SCBA)	☐
3	Supplied air systems (SABA)	☐
3	Full body harnesses	☐
6	Hard hats	☐
6	Pairs leather gloves	☐
6	Safety glasses	☐
1	Basket stretcher	☐
1	Reeves Sleeve®	☐
1	Backboard	☐
	Quick energy food & drink	☐
1	Propane heater with extension tube	☐

Figure 1-30. Parkway checklist.

Response

RECEIVING THE ALARM
The Role of the Dispatcher
Gathering and Transmitting Information
The One-Call System for Locating Utility Installations

RESPONDING TO THE ALARM
The Rescue Vehicle Driver's Role
Factors That Affect Response
Alternate Routing

PARKING AT THE ACCIDENT SITE
Factors to Consider When Parking the Rescue Unit

KNOWLEDGE OBJECTIVES

The rescuers should be able to—

☑ Define relevant words and phrases
☑ Summarize activities of the response phase of a trench rescue operation
☑ Describe the role of the emergency service dispatcher in a trench rescue operation
☑ List at least eleven bits of information that a dispatcher should elicit from a person who is reporting a trench accident
☑ Describe the one-call system for locating utility installations and relate the value of the system to a trench rescue effort
☑ Describe the roles and responsibilities of an emergency vehicle driver
☑ List at least seven factors that may affect the response of an emergency vehicle to an accident scene
☑ Relate the danger of parking an emergency vehicle too near the immediate trench accident site
☑ List at least four factors that should be considered when parking an emergency vehicle at an accident scene

SKILL OBJECTIVES

The rescuer working individually or as part of a team should be able to—

☑ Elicit the proper information from the person who is reporting a trench accident
☑ Initiate a class for information from the local one-call system
☑ Drive the emergency vehicle safely to the accident site
☑ Park the vehicle in a safe place

Words and Phrases You May Be Seeing For the First Time

Bulldozer. A crawler-equipped machine with a large horizontal blade designed for land clearing, material moving, etc.

Community resource. A firm or other organization that can provide personnel, equipment, and machines at the time of an emergency.

Dewatering. Removing water from the work area.

Euphoria. A feeling of well-being or elation.

Front-end loader. A rubber tire or crawler-equipped machine with a movable bucket at one end.

Grade crossing. A railroad crossing at highway level.

Loam. A combination of sand and clay.

Mobile crane. A crane that is provided with rubber tires for over-the-highway travel.

One-call system. A service from which contractors, emergency service personnel, and others can obtain information on the location of underground utilities in any area.

Secondary cave-in. The collapse of another portion of a trench wall after the initial accident.

SOP. Standard operating procedure.

Staging area. A gathering point; in this case, for emergency service and support apparatus, equipment, and personnel.

Underground utilities. Conduits carrying water, gas, electric transmission lines, sewage, etc.

Wire span. The distance between utility poles.

The second phase of a rescue operation begins when a call for help is transmitted and ends when the rescue unit is parked safely at the scene of the incident. There are three distinct activities common to the response phase: receiving the alarm, responding to the alarm, and arriving at the scene. Dispatchers, emergency vehicle drivers, and rescue officers all play important roles in the response phase of a rescue operation.

RECEIVING THE ALARM

Suppose you receive word of George and Henry's accident like this:

> **Dispatcher:** "Meadowbrook Station, respond to an accident at the new Parkway Industrial Complex."

You will not know much about the call, will you? You will know that your unit is to respond, and you will know generally where to go, although the complex covers a half–square mile. But will you be responding to a vehicle accident, a structure collapse, or an accident during which someone has become trapped under a machine or dirt?

THE ROLE OF THE DISPATCHER

Dispatchers are a vital part of a community's emergency services system. They must realize that they may often play a pivotal role in the success or failure of a firefighting or rescue operation. Dispatchers must always keep in mind that someone may die if a call is not handled properly. A lawsuit could follow. Do not ignore the consequences of a poorly handled or bungled call for help.

Dispatchers must have a sense of priority. People who receive many calls in a short space of time in a large communications facility must be able to sort out and act upon calls that indicate a real threat to life. This is both an innate sense and a skill.

Dispatchers must be calm, and they must be able to calm others. A person who calls to report a fire or an accident usually is excited. It may be *his* house that is on fire, or it may be *her* child that has been injured in an accident. Becoming excited is a natural reaction to a crisis situation. By tone of voice and technique of questions, dispatchers can calm callers and prompt them for important bits of information.

Dispatchers must be resourceful. Having a standard operating procedure (SOP) is good, but having a dispatcher who can function effectively when the elements of an SOP cannot be brought together is even better. There are times when prescribed back-up units are not available and when specified com-

munity resource personnel cannot be located. When this happens, a resourceful dispatcher does not simply tell the requesting officer that a service is not available; he finds an alternative.

Dispatchers must be able to work under pressure. Like firefighting and rescue personnel, dispatchers never know whether the next call will be a routine one or the most important one of the year. If the call is for a unique emergency, a dispatcher must be able to simultaneously answer telephones; receive, act upon, and transmit radio messages; consult operations manuals; and perform other vital functions without becoming flustered.

Dispatchers must have both the knack and the tools for gathering and transmitting accurate and complete information.

GATHERING AND TRANSMITTING INFORMATION

In more progressive emergency service communications centers, dispatchers are not only trained to elicit certain facts from callers regarding emergency situations, they are also provided with special forms on which to record those facts. This helps provide a degree of certainty that fire and rescue officers will be provided with information that will help them make effective plans of action.

The form that is shown in Figure 2-1 might be used by a dispatcher to record details of a trench accident. Regardless of the form used, the following points should be covered.

THE LOCATION OF THE ACCIDENT

Recall the message that was quoted as a poor example of a dispatcher's communication skill. The message told rescue personnel nothing more than that there was an accident somewhere in the Parkway Industrial Complex. Even though the streets in the Parkway Complex have yet to be named, the dispatcher could have made an effort to determine that the accident site was located two blocks in and then to the right of MacArthur Drive, the main entrance to the complex.

In urban areas where streets have names and buildings have numbers, the dispatcher must be sure that the entire address is received and transmitted, along with the proper geographical designation if there is one (north, east, south, west). Furthermore, the dispatcher should ask the caller to pinpoint the address within a certain community or development if the street has a common name such as Market or Main Street.

In rural areas, determining the correct location of

TRENCH ACCIDENT REPORT

Time Received: _____ AM/PM   Name of the Contractor: _____   One-Call System Alerted: _____

Exact Location: _____

Phone Number: _____

Development: _____

City/Town: _____

Nature of Accident:

☐ Trench Cave-in

☐ Construction Equipment Involved

☐ Pipe/Boulder Entrapment   Location of Job Office Trailer: _____

☐ Other   Community Resources Alerted: _____

Number of Persons Involved: _____

Extent of Injuries: _____

Number of Persons Trapped: _____   Language Problems: _____

Status of the Caller: _____

Phone Number: _____   Special Problems: _____

Width & Depth of the Trench: _____

Soil Type: _____   Action Taken: _____

On the Scene Hazards:

☐ Wires Down

☐ Distrupted Underground Utilities

☐ Gas   Other Information: _____

☐ Water

☐ Electric   Companies Dispatched: _____   Time: _____

☐ Flammable Liquids

☐ Steam

☐ Caustics

☐ Radioactive Materials

☐ Chemicals

☐ Water (Ground)

☐ Deep-Well System   Special Units Dispatched: _____

☐ Well-Point System

☐ Exposed But Unbroken Utilities

☐ Other   Dispatcher: _____

Figure 2-1. Dispatch form.

an incident may be difficult. A caller may report that there has been a trench cave-in on Route 10 five miles south of town. If the caller cannot immediately be more precise about the location of the incident, the dispatcher should ask what crossroad is near the accident site, what place of business can be seen from the phone's location, or what mile marker the caller may have passed on the way to the phone. If the caller does not know any of these, the dispatcher should ask about visible landmarks such as a water tower, a radio antenna, or even a large silo. A name on a mailbox may be helpful. Even a number on a utility pole will provide a clue as to where the caller is. If the caller can provide absolutely no information as to the location of the accident, the dispatcher should ask the number of the telephone the caller is using. The telephone company can determine the location of a particular phone without delay.

THE NATURE OF THE ACCIDENT

It is not enough for a dispatcher to learn that "there has been an accident." He must learn the nature of the accident so that the proper emergency service units can be alerted. In a trench accident situation, the dispatcher should learn whether there has been a cave-in; he should learn also whether or not there is any heavy machinery involved in the accident. If he knows that a backhoe has tumbled into the excavation at the time of the cave-in, for example, he will be able to initiate calls for a mobile crane without delay.

THE NUMBER OF PEOPLE INVOLVED

When he knows how many people are involved in the accident, a dispatcher can make a judgment as to calling additional ambulances and rescue units right away.

PROBLEMS OF ENTRAPMENT AND INJURIES

Although it might seem unnecessary to ask whether or not people are trapped in a cave-in, the questions should be asked. Perhaps the one man who was in the trench at the time of the cave-in scrambled free just as the spoil pile slid into the excavation. At the same time, the dispatcher should query the caller about injuries so that responding units will be able to prepare for emergency care activities.

THE STATUS OF THE CALLER

If the caller is familiar with the job site, there are a great many more details that can be learned about a trench incident and passed on to the responding rescue officer.

If the dispatcher learns that the caller is merely a witness to the accident and is not connected with the construction activity in some way, he may simply take the caller's name and phone number, then

disconnect. Asking technical questions a caller cannot answer is pointless. If the dispatcher determines that the caller is part of the construction team, however, he should ask him to stay on the line while he alerts the appropriate emergency units. When he gets back to the caller, the dispatcher should attempt to obtain the following information.

THE WIDTH AND DEPTH OF THE TRENCH

If the dispatcher can learn the dimensions of the trench from the caller, this information can be passed on to the rescue officer. The officer will know immediately whether he can handle the situation with the equipment he is carrying on his rig or whether he will need assistance from community resource personnel.

THE TYPE OF SOIL

What sort of soil he will have to stabilize is an important detail for the rescue officer. If the soil is unmanageable, he will have to formulate a plan of action other than sheeting and shoring.

ON-THE-SCENE HAZARDS

The dispatcher should specifically inquire as to whether wires were brought down by poles that were dislodged by the earth shift. He should also ask about broken gas mains and other disrupted underground utilities. Responding rescuers can then be made aware of the hazards that may be a threat to their lives as well as the lives of people on the scene.

WATER HAZARDS

The dispatcher should ask whether water lines were broken when the trench wall collapsed. Again, he can initiate the prearranged response of dewatering equipment if he knows of a water problem.

THE NAME OF THE CONTRACTOR

If in his questioning the dispatcher has not learned the name of the contractor, he should ask now. He can then call the contractor's office and have a supervisor who is familiar with the job report to the scene.

LANGUAGE PROBLEMS

Asking whether everyone on the job site speaks English is not as unnecessary as it sounds. There are a great many construction sites in this country at which the majority of the crew members do not speak English. If the dispatcher determines that this is the case, he can locate a suitable interpreter from his community resource files.

Imagine how a dialogue might develop between your Center County Fire Department dispatcher and the person who is reporting George and Henry's plight.

Dispatcher	Caller
"Center County Fire Department. Do you have an emergency?"	"I sure do! There has been an accident at the new Parkway Industrial Complex."
"What sort of accident, sir?"	"A trench has caved in."
"Exactly where is the accident?"	"It's about half a block to the right of MacArthur Drive on the second street in from Bayard Parkway."
"What is your name, sir, and what number are you calling from?"	"What difference does that make? C'mon, man, people are trapped!"
"Please calm down, sir. I need the details so I can send help."	"OK. I'm John Edwards. I'm calling from 555-8374."
"How many people are involved, Mr. Edwards?"	"Two, as far as I know."
"Are they still in the trench?"	"Yes."
"Are they buried?"	"One is, and one's buried to his chest."
"Is there any heavy equipment involved in the accident?"	"No."
"Are there any injured persons outside the trench?"	"No."
"Mr. Edwards, are you associated with the job?"	"I'm the contractor."
"Will you please stay on the line? I am going to alert the rescue squad. Then I would like to get more details from you."	"OK."
(At this time, the dispatcher alerts the first-due emergency service units. He then returns to the caller.)	
"Sir, what is the width and depth of the trench?"	"It's 4 feet wide by about 12 feet deep."
"What is the type of soil?"	"It's clay and sand. It's a . . . uh . . . a loamy-type soil."
"Are there any downed wires or broken gas lines or any other hazards?"	"No."
"Is there any water in the trench?"	"No."
"Do all the crew members speak English?"	"Yes."
"Is there anything you can add that will be helpful to the rescue officer?"	"I can't think of anything."
"Thank you, Mr. Edwards. Will you watch for the rescue units and guide them to the scene?"	"OK. I'll meet them on MacArthur."

A wealth of detailed information was gathered by the dispatcher, and, according to the time clock, the information was logged in 75 seconds. With the first-response units alerted and on the way, the dispatcher can now pass on the details that will help the officer develop a rescue plan even before he arrives on the scene. The radio message that contains those facts might sound like this:

Dispatcher	Rescue 63
"Fire radio to Rescue 63."	"Go ahead, fire radio."
"I have additional information on the Parkway Incident. Can you copy, Rescue 63?"	"Go ahead, fire radio."
"The caller reports that two workmen are still in the trench, no heavy equipment is involved, and there are no apparent related hazards. The trench is 4 feet wide by 12 feet deep in sandy loam. OK, Rescue 63?"	"Message received, fire radio. Stand by for a community resource request."
"Standing by, Rescue 63."	

A few minutes after the call for help was placed, the rescue unit was on the way, the rescue officer was developing his plan of action from the details that were gathered by the dispatcher, and the dispatcher was ready to call upon a wide variety of community resources.

THE ONE-CALL SYSTEM FOR LOCATING UTILITY INSTALLATIONS

In many parts of the United States there is a unique service available to contractors who are preparing to make underground installations: the one-call system. This service is so important and so underutilized by the emergency services that we will describe it in detail.

The system includes a network of reporting centers from which contractors can learn the location of all underground utility installations such as water mains, sewer lines, and telephone cables, in the areas of their job sites. The service is made available in the interests of public service and safety and reducing customer service interruptions.

When a contractor plans to excavate, he may call a toll-free 800 number at least 2 days before beginning work. The operator at the message center asks a series of questions that will provide the center with the exact location of the proposed work site. Employees of the center locate the job site on a master map and determine the grid coordinates. The information that a contractor plans to dig at a certain location is sent via high-speed teletype to the participating utility providers—organizations that may have underground utility installations at the proposed dig site.

The service is quick. As soon as they are received, requests for information and grid coordinates are sent to participating members, who immediately locate the proposed job site on their grid maps. The utilities that make up the service must respond to the contractor's request for information by informing him that either they have no underground installations at the designated location, or that there are installations in the area and they are sending a crew to the site to mark the location of the utilities.

The utility company crews mark the location of underground installations with colored stakes, paint, or flags. Colors recommended by International One-Call Systems are: orange for communications, red for power, blue for water, green for sewer lines, yellow for gas, brown for other than potable water, purple for radioactive materials, and white for proposed excavation sites. When he sees colored markers on his job site, the contractor knows that "the system" has worked for him!

The cost of operating the one-call system is shared by the participating organizations according to their number of underground installations. Secondary parties are charged a fee according to the plant maintained.

The network of reporting centers is indispensable to the emergency services of this country. From one call placed through his communications center, a fire or rescue officer can be made aware of underground installations at scenes of trench cave-ins, building collapses, major fires, and other unique or large-scale emergencies. Moreover, he can avail himself of the services of experts sent to the scene by participating utility companies.

RESPONDING TO THE ALARM

Imagine again our hypothetical trench accident at the Parkway Industrial Complex.

You have a dedicated trench rescue unit that is on its way to the scene of the accident. You have been armed with information about the incident. But in order to begin the rescue operation, you must arrive safely. Safe arrival depends on the ability of the rescue vehicle driver.

THE RESCUE VEHICLE DRIVER'S ROLE

There are three parts to the driving effort. A rescue vehicle cannot make a safe response without a well-prepared and well-kept vehicle, a reasonably safe and properly maintained roadway, and a trained and responsible driver.

A rescue vehicle driver must be physically and mentally capable of operating his rig in a variety of situations. He should not have uncorrected vision problems, nor should he have any impairment that might disable him while he is driving to the scene of an emergency. He should not have any physical disability that will prevent safe operation of the vehicle. A rescue vehicle should not be operated by a driver who is taking medications that cause either drowsiness or euphoria, pain killers, or tranquilizers. And, most certainly, a rescue vehicle should not be driven by someone who is under the influence of alcohol or drugs.

Good mental condition is as important as good physical condition. A rescue vehicle operator should not be preoccupied with personal problems, nor should he drive if he is emotionally upset. He should have a healthy attitude toward his driving ability and other drivers using the road. He should have confidence but not a feeling of superiority. Moreover, a rescue vehicle operator should share a spirit of cooperation and mutual respect with the rescue officer. There should never be an argument as to where the vehicle should be parked at the emergency scene, nor should there be any discussion as to how personnel will be used. And, of course, the driver of a rescue vehicle must know, understand, and respect the laws that govern the operation of emergency vehicles in his state.

FACTORS THAT AFFECT RESPONSE

There are a number of factors that affect the response of emergency vehicles.

DAY OF THE WEEK

The day of the week has a direct bearing on the flow of traffic within any given area. Weekdays—from Monday through Friday—are the days of heaviest traffic because people are commuting to and from work. On a Saturday the flow of commuter traffic generally diminishes, but shopper traffic picks up around shopping centers. On a Sunday, traffic is usually minimal, although there may be temporary congestion around churches, and expressways may be packed in the late afternoon and evening with people returning home from a weekend vacation or a Sunday outing.

TIME OF THE DAY

Not too many years ago, daily traffic patterns were predictable. In the morning, vehicles moved from the suburbs to the cities, and in the afternoon, the flow was reversed as people went home. Today the situation is much different. With the advent of satellite bedroom communities, massive shopping centers, and huge industrial parks of office building complexes, traffic tends to flow over major roadways equally in both directions at any time. People from the suburbs are going to work in the cities, and people from the cities are going to work in the suburbs. From before 7 am to well after 6 pm, emergency vehicle drivers can anticipate packed roads, blocked intersections, and creeping traffic. In the areas around large shopping malls, these conditions can be expected to last until 9 pm or even later.

WEATHER

Rain and fog reduce driving speeds, and reduced speeds result in increased response times. Ice on the roads increases response times even more, and heavy snow sometimes temporarily prevents a response altogether.

DETOURS

Traffic can be severely slowed by road construction and maintenance, sewer installations, and building construction. Detours and lane restrictions may last for only a few hours, or they may be in force for months or even years. Often a detour affects the operation of emergency vehicles more than the closing of lanes on a multilane roadway. When several lanes merge into one, there is often no way for emergency vehicles to leave the road or for other vehicles to pull out of their way, and siren-sounding, light-flashing, and horn-blowing will be of little help.

RAILROADS

Although the replacement of grade crossings with bridges and underpasses has greatly reduced vehicle obstructions, traffic is still blocked occasionally by slow-moving freight trains, especially in rural areas. In small towns a long train can effectively halt the flow of traffic in all directions and even isolate part of the town.

BRIDGES AND TUNNELS

Bridges are built to allow the flow of traffic over natural dividers such as rivers and gorges. Tunnels are generally dug so that traffic can pass under bodies of water. Although bridges and tunnels usually aid the flow of vehicles, they are at times responsible for traffic jams.

SCHOOLS AND SCHOOL BUSES

Schools contribute to traffic slowdowns. The reduced speed limits that are in force during school hours can slow the flow of vehicles. Crossing guards who control traffic signals can disrupt the normal flow of traffic. There is also a natural tendency for drivers to slow down when they enter streets crowded with school children. School buses usually slow the flow of traffic, especially when the buses make frequent stops along a narrow roadway.

Emergency vehicle drivers should remember that the sight and sound of a fire truck, rescue unit, or ambulance attract children, who may venture out in the street to watch them pass by. Accordingly, every emergency vehicle should be slowed when it approaches a school or playground area during the daylight hours.

As you can see, the flow of traffic is affected by many conditions. The movement of a rescue vehicle will certainly be affected if the weather is bad, if there are detours, if the vehicle must pass over a crowded bridge, or if other limiting factors are present. If you are the officer on a vehicle that is having a problem responding to the scene of an accident, you should consider taking another route.

ALTERNATE ROUTING

Although the shortest distance between two points is always a straight line, the fastest way to get from one place to another may not be the most direct. You, as a rescue officer, must constantly monitor road conditions in your service area, and you must consider how changing conditions will affect emergency responses. Preplan maps should always show continuously troublesome traffic spots such as school zones, bridges, tunnels, and grade crossings. Maps should also show temporary problem areas, such as detours, construction sites, and other slowdown points. Drivers should be advised of changing road conditions at training sessions and driver meetings. Whenever possible, alternate routes should be established around both permanent and temporary impediments.

PARKING AT THE ACCIDENT SITE

Pulling up to the scene of a trench accident may be no different from arriving at the scene of a building fire or vehicle accident—if the run can be made entirely on a paved roadway. If the accident has occurred at a construction job site, however, you may have to drive for a considerable distance around equipment and piles of construction materials over roadways that are little more than muddy, rutted paths. As a matter of fact, at some job sites you may have to have your rig towed by a bulldozer; or you may have to leave the rig and have your heavy sheet-ing and shoring carried to the rescue site in the bucket of a front-end loader.

Let us say that when you respond to the Parkway Incident you can drive directly to the accident site even though the roads are unpaved. It is a hot day and there has been no rain for some time.

> **Remember**
> Under no circumstances should you simply pull up to the side of the excavation so that the rescue equipment will not have to be carried any distance. To do so may put you in a hazard zone. Also, the weight of your unit and its vibrations may cause a secondary collapse of the trench walls.

FACTORS TO CONSIDER WHEN PARKING THE RESCUE UNIT

Hazards should be your first consideration, and you must remember that both traffic and non-traffic hazards can make the work area unsafe.

TRAFFIC

Your rescue vehicle should not be parked by just placing it across the road. True, you will want to keep non-emergency vehicles away from the rescue scene, but blocking the road with your rig will also deny access to emergency and community resource vehicles that have been dispatched to help you. Other ways for directing traffic will be discussed in Phase 4—Hazard Control.

PROXIMITY TO HAZARDS

If your dispatcher has provided you with details of on-the-scene hazards while you were responding (or if someone runs up to you with this information as you arrive), temporarily park away from the danger zone until you can assess the situation yourself.

If wires are down, park at least one full span away from the span that is broken so there will be no chance that the wires will arc and whip toward your unit. If a gas leak has been reported, make every effort to park not only a safe distance away but also upwind, if possible.

Be wary about parking too close to the accident site if a water main has been broken by the trench collapse. Water flowing from a broken main can undermine the roadway for a considerable distance. You could find yourself in the embarrassing position of having your rescue vehicle lifted from a very large hole with a very large crane!

PROXIMITY TO THE TRENCH

If traffic and other hazards do not require parking away from the rescue site, approach the excavation with care. Again, apparatus should be positioned far enough away so that vibrations and the vehicle's weight will not contribute to a secondary cave-in. It is suggested that you park no closer than 50 feet from an open trench, even if the road is paved and you are reasonably sure of the condition of the ground beneath.

As you approach the rescue area, consider the surrounding ground, especially if the area is hilly. If there is ice on the road, or if the roadway is extremely slippery because of mud, there may be the added danger of sliding into the open trench if you park the rescue unit uphill from the trench. Always keep in mind the possibility of exhaust fumes entering the trench.

ACCESSIBILITY FOR OTHER VEHICLES AND EQUIPMENT

When you decide on a parking space, be certain that your unit will not block parking lots or uncluttered open areas that may serve as staging areas for other emergency vehicles or as equipment fabrication areas.

The response phase of a trench rescue operation involves a great deal more than simply jumping into the rescue vehicle, rushing to the scene, and screeching to a halt at the side of the open trench. From the time that the alarm is received until the time that you find a suitable place to park, you must consider—

- Details about the accident
- Factors that can affect response
- Factors that should influence the parking of the unit

THE PARKWAY INCIDENT—
RESPONSE

Jot down the information you've obtained about the Parkway Incident thus far:

The exact location? _____

_____

The nature of the emergency? _____

_____

The problems of entrapment and injury? _____

_____

Status of the caller? _____

_____

Width and depth of the trench? _____

Type of soil? _____

_____

On-the-scene hazards? _____

_____

Name of the contractor? _____

_____

Language problems? _____

_____

The alarm has been received and you are on the way. What units are responding? (Remember that you are responding to the Parkway Incident with the units that would normally respond from your real-life home station.) _____

_____

Open to the map in Appendix A. You will see that it is a fairly straight run from the Meadow-brook Station to the Parkway Industrial Complex. But there are some problem areas along the way that could delay or even halt your response. From the information contained on the map, what do see that could delay you? _____

_____

_____

Do you see any alternate routes that might be better if you do run into a problem along the main route? If so, how would you proceed? _____

_____

_____

You have arrived at the intersection of Bayard Parkway and MacArthur Drive, the entrance to the new Parkway Industrial Complex. Mark your location with an X on the site plan. Take a look at the site plan. How will you proceed to the rescue site? _____

_____

_____

Once on the rescue site, where will you have your units park? Remember the points made earlier about blocking the way for other emergency vehicles and about parking with regard for hazards and the unstable trench. Keeping these points in mind, draw the locations of your units on the site plan.

    With your units safely parked and your personnel standing by for your orders, you are ready to make an assessment of the situation. _____

_____

_____

Assessment

THE PRIMARY ASSESSMENT

Determining Who Is In Charge
Determining What Has Happened
Seeing If There Are Any Communication Barriers
Assessing Immediate Injury Problems
Looking for Hazards
Determining How Many People Are Buried
Determining Where the People Are Buried

THE SECONDARY ASSESSMENT

Assessing On-The-Scene Capabilities
Requesting Additional Resources
Assigning Personnel

KNOWLEDGE OBJECTIVES

The rescuer should be able to—

- ☑ Define relevant words and phrases
- ☑ Summarize activities of the assessment phase of a trench rescue operation
- ☑ List the steps of the primary assessment
- ☑ List at least ten hazards that may be present at the scene of a trench accident
- ☑ List at lease seven clues that may be useful when determining the location of a buried trench accident victim
- ☑ Describe the secondary assessment

SKILL OBJECTIVES

The rescuer should be able to—

- ☑ Conduct a primary and secondary assessment

WORDS AND PHRASES YOU MAY BE SEEING FOR THE FIRST TIME

Asphyxiant. A gas capable of causing death from oxygen deficiency.

Atmospheric monitor. A device used to analyze oxygen content, hydrocarbons, and toxic gases.

Batter boards. A series of horizontal boards spanning a trench, used by a contractor to set the line and grade of a pipe.

Bisect. To cross or intersect.

Cohesive. Holding together firmly.

Cut sheet. A job foreman's daily plan. Shows depth and grades for pipe.

Deep-well system. A means for dewatering the ground around a trench. In a line parallel to the trench, pipe casings with screens are driven into the ground to a level below that of the trench floor. Electric submersible pumps lowered into the casings continually dewater the work area. The water is collected and discharged at a point distant from the site.

Disrupted utilities. Broken water mains, gas mains, service lines, electrical conduits, etc.

Downed wires. Electric transmission lines brought down from utility poles by accident.

Engineer's hubs. Stakes placed on a utility construction job site by a layout crew. Symbols on the stakes tell the contractor where and how deep he should dig.

Exposed utilities. Gas mains, water mains, electrical conduits, etc., that are exposed but unbroken during a trench-digging operation.

Fissure. A narrow opening in the ground; a crack of some length and considerable depth.

Flag stake. A piece of lath with a colored ribbon attached to mark the location of an engineer's hub. The stake should bear information about the centerline and depth of the trench.

Gas main. Generally a large-diameter pipeline that carries natural gas under the streets.

Gas service line. A small-diameter pipe that connects the consumer with the gas main under the street.

Grade pole. A wood or fiberglass pole that is either cut to a certain length or provided with markings. It is used by workmen when they are setting pipes on grade.

Grease can and brush. A can of lubricant that is helpful for joining slip-joint pipe and the brush with which the lubricant is applied.

Header. A large-diameter pipe with inlets for suction hoses and a connection for the suction side of a pump.

Hydrostatic pressure. The force generated by a liquid.

Hyperactivity. Excessive activity.

Landfill. A collection point for trash and garbage. In a sanitary landfill the waste is buried between layers of earth.

Language bank. A community resource from which an interpreter can be obtained; usually run by a hospital or a governmental agency.

Laser target. A square or triangular plastic device used in conjunction with a laser instrument to set the line and grade of pipe.

Lower explosive limit. In a range of percentages, the point at which a mixture of flammable gas and air will not ignite because there is an insufficient concentration of the gas.

Manhole. An accessway to sewer pipes, an opening used for maintenance and inspection.

Methane gas. The chief component of natural gas; colorless, odorless, and flammable.

Offset. The distance (in feet) perpendicular from an engineer's hub to the pipeline.

Pipe string. Lengths of pipe laid parallel to the trench lip in preparation for being joined and buried.

Primary assessment. The initial determination of what has happened in an accident situation; the "size-up."

Profile. A job blueprint that shows sectional elevation.

Secondary assessment. A study to see whether or not on-the-scene capabilities are sufficient to cope with an emergency situation.

Story pole. See *Grade pole.*

String lines. Strings placed on one side of and parallel to the trench. Used to determine grade.

Trash pump. A centrifugal or diaphragm pump designed to move water that contains mud, stones, and other debris.

Tripping hazards. Debris, tools, equipment, and anything else that may cause a person to stumble at a construction site.

Unbroken utilities. Water mains, gas mains, electrical conduits, and pipelines that remain intact (although they may be exposed) during a trenching operation.

Upper explosive limit. In a range of percentages, the point at which a mixture of flammable gas and air will not ignite because there is not sufficient oxygen.

Water main. Generally a large-diameter water-carrying pipeline that is laid under the street.

Water service line. A small-diameter pipe that connects a consumer to the water main.

Well casing. A large-diameter pipe (12 inches) that is used in deep-well systems.

Well-point system. A series of pipes driven into the ground around a trench for the purpose of dewatering the work area. Water is drawn through the pipes, into a header, and finally into the suction side of a pump.

The third phase of a rescue operation begins when the rescue vehicle is safely parked and ends when the officer-in-charge has committed the squad members to hazard control activities.

During this period the officer makes a two-part determination. In the primary assessment he ascertains what has happened and how many people are involved. From observations made during the secondary assessment, the officer decides either that the rescue can be undertaken with the forces and equipment at hand or that personnel and equipment from community resource organizations is needed.

The rescue officer's ability to formulate an effective plan of action based on observations is important at all times during a rescue effort, but at no time is this ability more important than during the assessment phase. In a very short time—perhaps less than a minute—the officer must be able to perceive hazards that may threaten everyone and everything on the scene, determine the number of people that must be rescued, and locate them. Moreover, the officer must be able to determine whether the rescue can be accomplished with the forces and equipment at hand.

Imagine that you are at the Parkway Industrial Complex. Your vehicles are safely parked and the crew is standing by for orders. Before you give any orders, however, you must make assessments.

THE PRIMARY ASSESSMENT

There are two ways in which you can assess an accident situation. You can run around helter-skelter (and cast doubt on your ability) or you can make your assessment in a calm and orderly manner (and inspire confidence).

You must walk from where your unit is parked (Point A) to the side of the trench (Point B), so why not do more than simply walk from Point A to Point B and make the trip a learning experience? You can use your powers of observation to perceive hazards as you walk. As you start out with a wide field of vision, look for the hazards most distant from the trench. As you approach the opening, look for hazards that are closer. Then, when you arrive at the lip of the opening, look for hazards that may be present in the trench. You will note that the steps of the primary assessment are arranged in just that order.

Before you leave the rescue unit and your crew, however, determine who is in charge of the workers who have met with the accident.

DETERMINING WHO IS IN CHARGE

It would be unusual to arrive at the scene of any sort of accident and not have at least one person run up and present a detailed (and in some cases, gruesome) account of what has happened. More often than not, a rescue officer is set upon by a number of people—all knowledgeable of the accident, all clamoring to be heard, and all more than happy to give their advice as to how the situation might best be handled. You can surely expect this to be the case at the scene of a trench accident.

Instead of trying to sort out facts from the accounts of several individuals, simply ask, "Who is in charge here?" When that individual steps forward, take him aside. Ask him to have his workmen congregate at a location just out of the danger zone. It is important that they stay together. Equipment operators may be needed to operate cranes or earth-moving machinery during the rescue operation, and laborers may be needed to move sheeting and shoring and to relieve rescuers during the digging effort. While the foreman is instructing his workmen, have squad members gently move spectators to a safe area away from the rescue equipment.

Ask the foreman to stay with you during the rescue operation. Unless you are construction-oriented, you should welcome the company of an individual who can supplement your knowledge of rescue procedures with his knowledge of construction practices.

Remember
When you arrive on the scene and are besieged by people urging you into action and offering advice, do not become the typical authoritarian. Throwing your weight around and ordering people about in a discourteous way will do nothing but create hostility, especially among the workmen. If and when you need them during the rescue operation, you may be given some rather unpleasant suggestions, including one that is both anatomically and physiologically impossible.

Now, somewhat isolated from the crowd and ready to walk to the trench, you should turn to the foreman and determine exactly what has happened.

DETERMINING WHAT HAS HAPPENED

What you need at this point are facts about the accident. What you do not need is a dissertation. If the foreman inclines toward a prolonged description of the event, gently steer him away with some simple questions. How many people are buried? How long have they been buried? Is anyone outside the trench hurt?

If you learn that a number of people are buried (as might be the case when large-diameter pipe is being laid in a deep trench), or that a number of people have been hurt, you can request additional EMS units right away.

If this is not the case, store what facts you are able to get from the foreman in your mind so that you can recall them as you continue your assessment.

SEEING IF THERE ARE ANY COMMUNICATION BARRIERS

As mentioned in the section on response, it may seem silly to think of an interpersonal communication problem at the scene of a trench accident. There are, however, a large number of non-English-speaking construction crews working throughout the country today.

Check with the foreman to see if any of the key witnesses do not speak English. You may want to ask such persons important questions during your assessment; consequently, you must be able to communicate with them. If you do find that a witness does not speak English, call your dispatcher right away. Have him check his community resource file for an appropriate interpreter. This will present no problem if you have the number of the closest language bank in your preplan. In addition to locating an interpreter, the dispatcher can probably arrange to have a police car quickly transport the person to the scene.

ASSESSING IMMEDIATE INJURY PROBLEMS

Look for injured workmen away from the trench. Someone may have been struck by a piece of equipment when the trench wall collapsed or may have been injured in a successful attempt to scramble out of the trench.

If you see that someone has been injured, or if the foreman tells you of an injured workman, alert the emergency medical personnel on the scene. Let them care for the injured; your responsibility is to continue the assessment.

If they are congregated where you can see them, glance quickly at the workmen. Look for signs of emotional distress in particular. Hyperactivity is a sign. Look for the person who is running around, waving his arms, exhorting rescuers to help his comrades. Listlessness is another sign. Look for persons who are sitting quietly and staring vacantly into space. Call the attention of the emergency medical personnel to these people; they may be in shock. If you see that a number of people need medical attention, call the communication center for more ambulances.

If the dispatcher has been trained to elicit information from callers in unique accident situations, you will be made aware of on-the-scene hazards while you are responding. Hearing about hazards during the response phase is helpful, but at the scene you must determine the hazards yourself.

LOOKING FOR HAZARDS

Remember that a variety of hazards can be caused by the collapse of a trench. Some may be little more than a nuisance; others can pose a very real threat to life and property. Remember, too, that while the threat may not be immediately evident, a trench rescue operation can be severely endangered by the following factors.

TRAFFIC

The danger of vehicles passing close to an unstable trench is twofold. The weight of cars and trucks can produce forces that will cause unsupported trench walls to collapse. Vehicles do not have to be right next to the trench to pose a threat, however. Given certain ground conditions, vibrations caused by vehicles 100 feet or more away can trigger a secondary collapse.

Many times traffic on the job is overlooked. Scrapers, bulldozers, and similar heavy equipment working at the site create tremendous vibrations which can affect the rescue effort. Other vibratory problems can be caused by trains and helicopters. On-site machinery can be shut down immediately. Such may not be the case with trains. If the cave-in occurs near active tracks send radio-equipped persons a mile up the tracks in both directions. Instruct them to notify you when a train is approaching. Until the trench is properly sheeted and shored, do not allow rescuers to work at the trench lip while the trains are passing. Once the trench is secure, it is still a good idea to keep the radio-equipped persons posted where they can let you know of oncoming trains so that you and your men will not go into cardiac arrest when a train rumbles through.

For helicopters, have your dispatcher call the nearest airport tower and have a restricted air space declared over the location of the incident. Do not underestimate the vibratory powers of "chopper" blades on a hot, humid day. Press helicopters can land at a safe distance and cover the story by land.

SPECTATORS

Uncontrolled bystanders can be both at risk and dangerous at the scene of a trench accident. People can fall into the opening in the ground when natural curiosity makes a crowd edge closer and closer to the center of attraction. The weight of a group of spectators—even one or two—may be all that is needed to cause an undermined shelf of earth to break away and drop into the trench. Because they may get in the way of rescuers and other emergency service personnel, bystanders must be described collectively as a hazard.

DOWNED WIRES

Trenches often are opened in or adjacent to roadways lined with utility poles. When the collapse of a trench wall extends for a considerable distance to the side (as is often the case when the soil is sandy), utility poles can become dislodged. Sometimes a dislodged pole remains upright, supported by unbroken wires. But more often than not the moving pole creates a pull on the wires sufficient for them to break, and the wires and the pole come down.

When wires are down at an accident site, the danger zone extends for a full unbroken span in both directions, and to the sides for as far as the broken wires would reach if fully extended. A utility pole can support primary and secondary power lines and a variety of other conductors, including telephone lines, fire alarm cables, cable television–transmission lines, and street light circuits. Any or all of these wires may carry the highest voltage if they come in contact with the primary power conductor.

WELL-POINT SYSTEM

A utility contractor cannot merely open the ground, lay pipes, and close the trench when the ground is wet and sandy. He must remove as much water from the ground as he can. Then he must make the trench safe in one of a number of ways. Dewatering with a well-point system is a popular technique (Figure 3-1).

A well-point system includes a series of pipes sunk into the ground parallel to the trench until their ends are below the level of the bottom of the trench. The pipes are spaced 3 to 10 feet apart and are connected to the suction inlet of a large pump. The pump then sucks water from the ground.

Finding a well-point system at the scene of a trench accident should alert you to the possibility of two hazardous conditions. The first results if the system is in operation. So much water can be removed by a well-point system that soil particles are no longer cohesive—they no longer stick together. Therefore, unsupported walls can be quite unstable. The second hazardous condition results if the system has been inoperative for a period of time. Un-

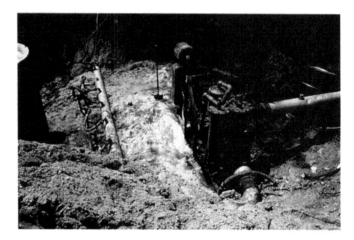

Figure 3-1. Well-point system.

supported trench walls can become saturated when the dewatering process stops. Hydrostatic pressure causes the walls to become unstable and collapse.

DEEP-WELL SYSTEM

When a trench must be opened in an extremely wet area, a contractor may be obliged to use the deep-well procedure for dewatering the ground before opening the trench. Well casings are bored into the ground next to where the opening will be made. An electrically powered submersible pump is lowered into each casing, and the casings then become wells. The discharge line carries water away from the job site (Figure 3-2).

As with the well-point system, hazardous conditions can result when trench walls are left unsupported. Dry walls caused by the dewatering procedure can crumble and collapse, and when the pumps are turned off the trench can become flooded.

Be aware that the very components of both systems can be a threat to rescuers as well. Headers, discharge lines, power cables, and exposed well cas-

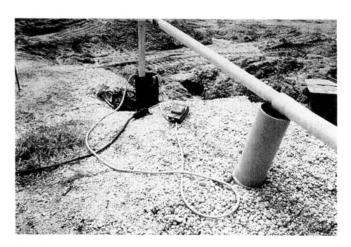

Figure 3-2. Deep well system.

ings can become tripping hazards, and power cables may cause electrocution if they are accidentally severed or submerged.

TRIPPING HAZARDS

All construction sites have a variety of tripping hazards. The ground around an open trench may be cluttered with batter boards, string lines, pallets, lengths of pipe, tools, lumber, or other equipment.

Once you are at the side of the trench you will be able to assess the threats of other hazards.

DISRUPTED UTILITIES

We have mentioned the problem of downed power lines. Be aware that not all power lines are suspended from utility poles. In many residential developments, office building campuses, and industrial parks, electric services are provided through buried conduits for aesthetic as well as practical reasons. Previously installed conduits can be found running parallel to or bisecting a newly dug trench. In either case, conduits can be severed when a trench wall collapses.

Electrical conduits are not the only supply lines that can be disrupted in a trench accident, however. In residential areas you can find gas mains and gas service lines, water mains and water service lines, and sewer lines broken by shifting earth. In industrial areas you may have a rescue problem compounded not only by broken water, gas, and sewer lines but also by broken fuel, oil, and gasoline supply lines, chemical pipelines, high-pressure steam lines, and even pipes carrying radioactive materials.

FLAMMABLE LIQUIDS

Fuel lines may be broken in a trench accident. If you can see or smell a flammable liquid in a trench, immediately call for the appropriate fire equipment response. Don't wait for the hazard control phase of the rescue operation. True, the flammable substance would be contained by the trench, but rescuers and victims would be in immediate danger throughout the entire rescue effort.

METHANE GAS

Regardless of where a trench accident may occur—in urban or rural areas—you must consider the problem of methane gas. Methane is the chief component (75 to 95 percent) of natural gas. It is a colorless, odorless, lighter-than-air gas that can seep into an open trench in several ways.

Marsh gas (another name for methane) is a by-product of the bacterial decomposition of vegetable **matter** that is underwater. The gas follows fissures in the ground, and if a trench is dug in a low-lying area along a river bank or lake front, or in a seashore

meadowland, gas-carrying fissures may terminate in a trench wall.

Methane also is generated in raw sewage and in the sludge that results from sewage treatment procedures. Because it is lighter than air, the gas drifts into the sewer system and finally into the trench if a sewer line is broken during a trench accident.

Methane gas is generated in landfills. When a trench is opened in ground that is directly over a landfill (as is often the case in new developments), methane seeps up into the trench from below.

The problem of methane generation is not a small one. Enough methane can be generated in one landfill to satisfy the gas needs of a small city for years.

Regardless of its source, methane gas poses a dual threat to rescuers at the scene of a trench accident. Methane is flammable—its lower explosive limit and upper explosive limit in air, respectively, are 5.3 percent and 31.9 percent. Because it is lighter than air, the concentration of gas and air in an open trench will seldom create a risk of explosion. Methane will burn vigorously at the bottom of a trench, however, much like vapors burn at the mouth of a fuel tank. Imagine the plight of a workman buried up to his chest and unable to move when methane that is seeping from the ground all around him is ignited.

Moreover, methane gas is an asphyxiant, and even though it is lighter than air it can affect rescuers who are required to work in still-air conditions in a trench.

> ## Remember
> Methane gas is colorless and odorless. Lack of a visible gas cloud or characteristic odor does not mean that methane gas is not present in an open trench.

EXPOSED BUT UNBROKEN UTILITIES

During your assessment you may look into a trench and see exposed but unbroken conduits and pipes. If the conduit or pipe bisects the trench it was probably uncovered by the contractor during the digging operation. If it appears in a void caused by either the collapse of the trench lip or loss of a section of the wall, it likely was exposed during the accident.

An unbroken conduit or pipe is dangerous because it could be broken during the rescue operation. The ground in the bottom of the trench would then be energized or flooded with whatever the pipe is carrying: flammable liquid or gas, water, or sewage.

Be aware that polyethylene or polypro gas pipe carries and stores tremendous volumes of static electricity. You can drain this off by draping a wet rag over the pipe and extending it to the ground. Keep it wet! Each exposed section of pipe must be treated independently.

FLOWING WATER

Water flowing from a broken main can, of course, drown a workman who is trapped in the trench. Flowing water also can cause the trench walls to collapse, and it can seriously undermine roadways for a considerable distance.

During the primary assessment, you should be able to identify obvious and non-obvious hazards to life and property.

In the Parkway Incident, your assessment for hazards reveals that the only threat to the rescue operation comes from an exposed water main that bisects the 4- by 12- by 25-foot-long trench. An 8-inch main is flowing at about 19,000 gallons per minute with a pressure of 100 psi. If the main breaks during the rescue effort, water will fill the trench in only 24 seconds!

At this point, you know whether there are hazards, but you have not completed your assessment. You still have to determine (if you have not yet been able to learn) how many people are buried, where they are buried, and whether you can get them out with the forces and equipment immediately available. Nonetheless, you can put some of your squad members to work. Some can be assigned to traffic and crowd tasks while others make the equipment ready for the sheeting, shoring, and digging operations.

Do not instruct rescuers or workmen to pick up items around the trench that you might have identified as tripping hazards. You may have to consider the position of some of these items as clues to the exact location of buried persons.

DETERMINING HOW MANY PEOPLE ARE BURIED

If there was an eyewitness to the accident, or if a workman was able to escape being buried, ask either of them how many workmen were in the trench at the time of the accident. If no one is sure of the number, go to where the workmen are assembled. Ask them to see who is missing. If they are not sure, have the foreman match each person to his time card or time book.

In the Parkway Incident, George is trapped by dirt up to his chest, but he is conscious and, although he is visibly upset, he is coherent. He tells you that only he and Henry were in the trench at the time of the accident and that Henry didn't get out in time. Because his arms are free, toss a helmet to George immediately. Any victims must be protected from falling objects early on. For those with only

their heads unburied, slide a panel into the trench lean-to fashion to protect them until you can sheet and shore. Do this after placing ground pads. Talk to them all the while, letting them know what you are doing.

DETERMINING WHERE THE PEOPLE ARE BURIED

If only a small section of the spoil pile or wall has slid into the trench—perhaps a section that is no more than 5 or 6 feet—you can be sure that anyone buried in the trench is under that relatively small mound of earth. On the other hand, when you see that a 20- or 30-foot section of the spoil pile or wall has slid into the trench, you know that locating the buried person or persons may be difficult. You could make the trench safe and simply start to dig, but you might start to dig at the wrong end of the mound of earth.

As in providing details concerning how many people have been involved in a trench accident, an eyewitness is the best source of information as to where victims are buried. Note the term "eyewitness." This means someone who was either in the trench when the accident occurred, or someone who actually observed the accident. There may not always be an eyewitness. No one in the trench may have been able to jump clear as the dirt slid in. No one may have been standing at the side of the trench watching the workmen when the accident happened. The backhoe operator may not have been in his machine when the pile slid or the wall collapsed. The fact that there is no eyewitness does not mean that you will have to dig blindly, however. There may be indicators as to the whereabouts of buried workmen, both in- and outside the trench.

CLUES THAT SHOULD BE CONSIDERED

Many "tripping hazards" could serve as valuable clues to the location of buried victims.

The pipe string. Most utility contractors have their workmen lay (or string) sections of pipe end to end next to where the trench will be dug and opposite to where the spoil will be piled (Figure 3-3). As each section of pipe is driven home, a new section is lowered into the trench. A good place to start looking for buried workmen is at the point in the trench that is in line with the end of the last pipe in the string. If they were following usual practices, the workmen will be somewhere between the end of the last length and the point at which it is joined to the preceding length. The next pipe to go in the trench is usually pointing to the victim.

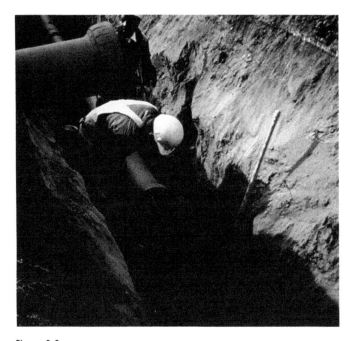

Figure 3-3. Pipe string.

A grease can and brush. It is sometimes necessary to use a lubricant when joining pipes. If so, workmen often scoop out a ledge in the trench wall to hold the grease can while they are driving home the sections. If you see a gallon can of grease with a paint brush in it resting on a ledge (Figure 3-4), you can be reasonably sure that the can marks the end of the pipeline, or at least the last section of pipe.

A laser target. If a laser device is being used to check the grade of a pipeline, workmen will often stick the laser target into the side of the trench wall when it is not needed. This, too, may indicate the end of the pipe and possibly the location of the workmen (Figure 3-5).

Laser targets are generally made of red or green plastic. When pipes are less than 18 inches in diameter, laser targets are usually round or triangular. When pipes are larger than 18 inches, the targets are usually rectangular.

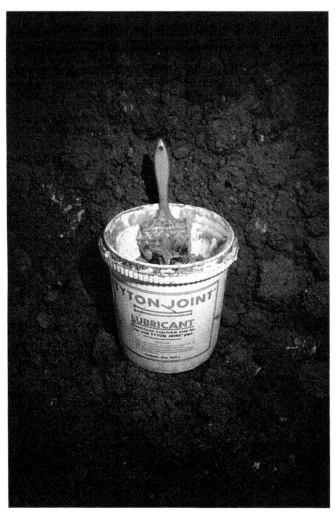

Figure 3-4. Grease can and brush.

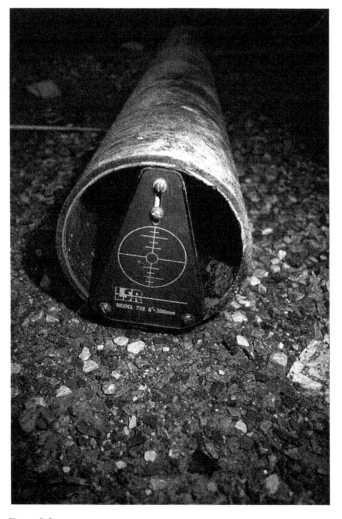

Figure 3-5. Laser target.

The grade pole. Also called the "story" pole, this is a graduated wood or fiberglass pole used in conjunction with a transit to determine grade. A grade pole sticking out of the ground will often signal the end of the pipeline, and possibly the location of the buried workmen (Figure 3-6). In this regard, a grade pole may often be viewed as a potential grave marker.

"Cat" or tire tracks. On many job sites the contractor is required to bed pipe with sand or stone. The bedding material is usually carried in the bucket of a tracked or wheeled loader, dumped into the trench, and spread by workmen with shovels. "Cat" or tire tracks at a right angle to the trench may indicate where the bedding material was dumped. Remember that the workmen may have been spreading the sand or stone from that point when the accident occurred.

Sounds in the pipe. If a spoil pile slides or a trench wall collapses while he is working with a pipe that is greater than 24 inches in diameter, an experienced workman may have the presence of mind to dive into the open end of the pipe. If he is lucky, he may be able to crawl completely into the pipe before the end is covered. At least he may be able to have his upper body protected by the pipe.

When you are on an accident scene where large-diameter pipe is being used, instruct a rescuer to go to the last manhole or catch basin and try to communicate with a possible survivor by shouting into the pipe. Have him listen for sounds of life; sounds travel for a considerable distance in a pipe. Tell him to shine a bright light into the pipe in an effort to see a trapped workman. With regard to respiratory protection, the rescuer must treat the manhole or catch basin as a confined space.

Profile and cut sheets. Profile sheets are actually blueprints of the job site, and cut sheets show the contractor how far he must dig to be able to lay the pipe at the correct depth and grade. The job foreman may have both profile sheets and cut sheets with him. When there are no other clues to the location of buried workmen, ask the foreman if he can determine their location from these documents. He will be able to tell you the maximum depth, at least.

Engineer's hubs. You may find yourself in a situation where the spoil pile slide or wall collapse is so extensive that the outline of the trench is virtually obliterated. When this is the case, do not have your rescuers dig blindly. Determine the centerline of the trench in one of a number of ways.

If a section of the pipe remains exposed, you can determine the centerline of the trench (even though you cannot see its edges) by sighting from the ex-

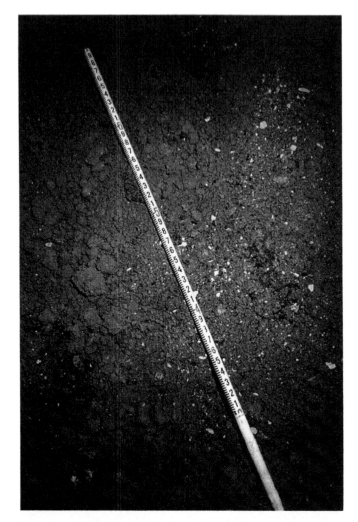

Figure 3-6. Grade pole.

posed pipe to the last manhole or catch basin. If there is no exposed pipe, sight from the backhoe to the last set manhole; and if the backhoe has been moved, stand between the tire or "cat" tracks and sight to the last manhole or catch basin. Some contractors lay down a trail of lime for the backhoe operators to follow while digging a trench. You can determine the centerline of a filled-in trench by sighting down this white line.

If you cannot determine the centerline of the trench by any of these methods, look for the engineer's hubs, which will indicate not only the centerline of the trench, but also the depth. An engineer's hub is usually a 2- by 2-inch stake that is driven almost to ground level anywhere from 10 to 25 feet from the trench. There is a tack driven into the center of the stake. Hub locations are marked with a flag stake that is usually 36 inches long and made from a piece of lath. A brightly colored ribbon or a piece of engineer's tape is generally tied to the upper end of the flag stake, and the color often designates the hub's purpose (for an offset, for a manhole, etc.)

Information about the trench is generally printed

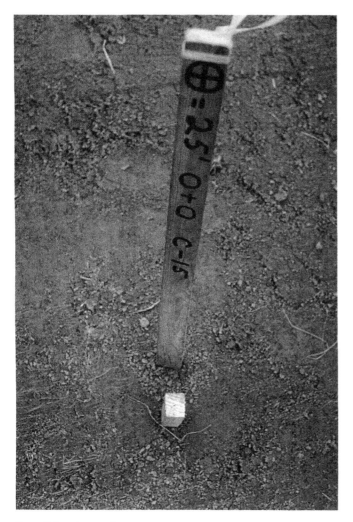

Figure 3-7. Flag stake.

on the flag stake with either a yellow crayon or a marker. Observe the flag stake shown in Figure 3-7. The symbol ⊕ represents the centerline of the manhole. The marking "25" means that the centerline of the manhole is 25 feet from the tack of the engineer's hub. The Marking "C-15" indicates that the trench is 15 feet deep; "C-15" is an instruction for the backhoe operator to cut, or dig, 15 feet. This measurement is determined from the tack on the engineer's hub. Other symbols that you might find on engineer's hubs and flag stakes are "MH," which stands for manhole, and "₵," which stands for the centerline of the trench.

Note that the terms "usually" and "generally" are used when discussing engineer's hubs and flag stakes. These hub and flag arrangements and markings shown are standard; however, not every contractor follows this practice exactly. It would be wise for you to find out how utility contractors mark engineer's hubs and flag stakes in your area.

As you can see, you do not have to rely solely on an eyewitness to determine where a trench accident victim is buried. There can be many clues, some ob-

vious, some that you will have to look for. When you are aware of whatever hazards may be present, and when you have determined the number and approximate location of the victims, then you can proceed.

THE SECONDARY ASSESSMENT

During the second part of the assessment phase of operations you must decide whether you can complete the rescue with the manpower and equipment at hand, or whether you will have to call for help. Your decision, of course, will be based on observations that you were able to make during your walk from the rescue unit to the side of the trench.

ASSESSING ON-THE-SCENE CAPABILITIES

Determine what resources you have on hand and what personnel you have available to use them.

SUPPLIES AND EQUIPMENT

Depending on the situation, you may need any or all of the following supplies and equipment:

- **Hazard control equipment.** Traffic cones, flags and flares; high-visibility ropes for crowd control activities; a lineman's clamp stick and glove set or a synthetic-fiber, weighted throwing line; and fire suppression equipment (if there are flammable substances present).
- **Dewatering equipment.** A portable pump (either gasoline or electrically powered) and discharge hoses. A trash or mud pump is preferred.
- **Air-moving equipment.** Either a smoke ejector, a utility blower, or a laser blower, preferably with an extension tube. Air lines from a wheeled compressor will suffice if a portable fan unit is not available (Figure 3-8).
- **Atmospheric monitoring equipment.** A go/no-go

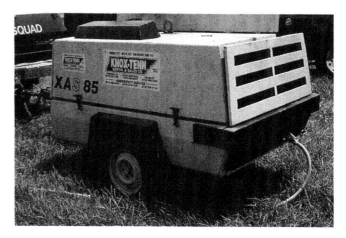

Figure 3-8. Air compressor.

system that gives you readings of oxygen content, hydrocarbons, and hydrogen sulphide. Readings should be taken every few minutes.

- **Lighting equipment.** A generator, power cables and distribution boxes, and portable floodlights. Battery-powered hand lights will be useful in the trench.
- **Tools.** A variety of power and hand tools.
- **Sheeting.** Shorform® panels or plywood sheets; 2- by12-inch uprights (either bolted to the panels or carried with them); and a supply of nuts, bolts, and washers.
- **Shoring devices.** Timbers, mechanical screw jacks, or pneumatic shoring in the sizes and numbers proper for the trench.
- **Patient transfer equipment.** A basket stretcher or other patient-carrying devices that can be lifted both vertically and horizontally; ropes, webbing, or straps for securing the patient; and a bridle or short lengths of rope for securing the stretcher to a lifting device.
- **Lifting equipment.** Used when ground conditions appear dangerous. A machine that can be placed a safe distance from the trench (such as a crane or an aerial ladder, platform, or tower) (Figure 3-9), to be used for lifting sheeting, walers, and other heavy material, and as an anchor point for man-lifting devices.
- **Earth-moving equipment.** A front-end loader, a backhoe, or a bulldozer.
- **Ladders.** Fire service—grade 24-foot extension ladders and a short ladder for climbing into and out of the trench.
- **Supplies.** Ropes, nails, scabs, wedges, and odd lengths of lumber.

Having the necessary supplies and equipment at the scene of a trench accident does not mean that you can conclude the rescue operation quickly and

efficiently. Trained, skilled people, and enough of them, are crucial to the success of your rescue operation.

MANPOWER

Many tasks can be accomplished by the same rescuer or teams of rescuers. For example, two squad members assigned to initial traffic control efforts can be reassigned when police officers arrive on the scene. Rescuers who are given the job of moving a downed wire can be assigned to sheeting and shoring tasks once they have moved the wire to a safe place. Squad members who put a portable pump in operation can be assigned to digging tasks, and so on.

It is impossible to say how many rescuers will be needed at the scene of a trench accident. You have to take each situation as it comes, and consider manpower needs in light of the tasks that must be accomplished.

If you respond with a special rescue unit, a truck company, and an ambulance, as in our hypothetical incident, you will probably have nine or ten rescuers available. If you are the rescue officer for a large volunteer fire department that has no daytime workforce problem, you may have more people than you need. On the other hand, if you are an officer in a municipal fire department that is short-handed, you will have to call for additional personnel from truck and engine companies.

Don't rely too heavily on using members of the construction crew. The average pipe-laying crew consists of a foreman, a backhoe operator, a loader operator, and three laborers. If two of the laborers are buried in the trench (as are George and Henry), the available manpower pool is reduced to four. The foreman should accompany you throughout the operation, so the pool is reduced to three. These three may be of no help because of anger, grief, or shock. Do not allow the backhoe operator to return to his machine. If you must dig, get another operator.

Whatever the situation, don't underestimate the need for manpower. It is unlikely that just a few squad members will be able to carry the heavy sheeting and shoring devices, manhandle them into the trench during the stabilizing efforts, and then go on to move a ton or more of dirt. If you find that you lack equipment or personnel, you will need to request more.

REQUESTING ADDITIONAL RESOURCES

Put yourself in the following situations:

Your fire department has such a refined SOP that calls for assistance require no more than the word "Help!" You are the officer-in-charge at the scene of a fire in a several-story building. The building is

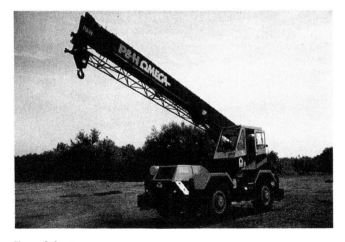

Figure 3-9. Crane.

fully involved. You see that the first-alarm companies will not be able to contain the fire, let alone extinguish it. You only have to pick up the radio microphone and call "Help" and the dispatcher will sound the second alarm for additional engine and truck companies.

Now you are the officer-in-charge at the scene of a serious motor vehicle accident. You feel that you cannot provide adequate emergency care and transportation for the several injured people with the personnel and equipment at hand. You only have to pick up the radio microphone and call "Help" and the dispatcher will send you additional ambulances.

But what will a dispatcher send to a rescue officer who needs help at the scene of a unique accident, such as a trench collapse, if he hears nothing more than "Help"? Fire equipment? Aerial apparatus? Ambulances? Squads? A quick response with the proper equipment to the scene of a trench accident requires that the officer-in-charge make a clear and concise request and that the dispatcher have at his fingertips all of the sources for people and items that might be needed.

Do not be vague when you call for help. If you need the services of a specialist, state clearly who you need and why, if possible. Thus the specialist can respond armed with information just as you were able to do.

> "Rescue 63 to radio. Have the water department respond to shut off an 8-inch main at this location."

If you need a particular piece of equipment, ask for it specifically:

> "Rescue 63 to radio. I need a trash pump to dewater the trench."

If you ask just for a pump, the dispatcher might send you the wrong type, or you and he might have to spend valuable minutes discussing your need over the radio.

If you need people to help, make your request in this manner:

> "Rescue 63 to radio. Send additional manpower to the scene."

The dispatcher will probably honor your request according to the department SOP in this case and send the next-due engine and/or truck company.

However, as detailed and correct as your request may be, help may be a long time in coming if the dispatcher does not have a list of community resources close at hand. In the same way that dispatch centers maintain resource lists for major fires, natural disasters, unique transportation accidents, radiological emergencies, and a host of other emergency situations, they should have a resource list for trench accident situations. Such a list can be maintained in a computer bank, on a microfilm, or on a sheet of notebook paper!

A sample community resource list is shown in Figure 3-10. Note that it contains just about every service and special piece of equipment that might be needed for a trench rescue operation. Also note that there are spaces for alternate sources of service and equipment. You can be sure that at least one or two primary sources will not be accessible when needed, and the last thing that a dispatcher needs at the time of an emergency is to have to leaf through the Yellow Pages.

ASSIGNING PERSONNEL

With your assessment complete and help on the way, you draw to a close the third phase of the rescue operation. Initial personnel assignments must be made according to priority. Give detailed instructions to rescuers (or other emergency service personnel, or even apparently-capable bystanders) for directing traffic until police officers can take over. Assign rescuers the tasks of neutralizing immediate hazards (such as downed wires and water in the trench). Ask some of the workmen to assist with the laying out of rescue equipment; the rescue unit driver can act as a sort of supply sergeant and direct their efforts. If other workmen are available, ask them to clear debris from the rescue area. Have rescuers prepare to ventilate the trench. Use the manpower at hand to launch the next phase of activity—hazard control.

COMMUNITY RESOURCES					
ITEM	SOURCE	HOURS	PHONE	CONTACT	HOME PHONE
			(800)		
One-Call system	Miss Utility of Delmarva	7:30 am/5 pm	282-8555	Mel Wyatt	594-0800
Timbers, uprights,	Martin Lumber Co.	8:00 am/5 pm	555-2400	Art Reid	821-3226
plywood	Beasley Building Supply	8:00 am/5 pm	555-7200	Bob Kalsch	555-4370
Shoring: pneumatic	Meadowood Water Dept.	8:00 am/6 pm	555-7100	Tom Holmbeck	597-0220
& hydraulic	Meadowood Sewer Authority	8:00 am/4:30 pm	555-7000	Bob Murray	594-3250
Shorform panels	Tidewater Utility Contr.	7:00 am/5 pm	584-2300	Harry Mellon	653-1301
	Rapposelli Construction	7:00 am/5 pm	555-4200	Joe Rapposelli	798-4491
	R. Tomasetti & Son	7:00 am/5 pm	584-3226	Ray Tomasetti	571-2630
Pumps: gas &	Meadowood Water Dept.	8:00 am/6 pm	555-7100	Tom Holmbeck	597-0220
electric	Meadowood Sewer Authority	8:00 am/4:30 pm	555-7000	Bob Murray	594-3250
	Tidewater Utility Contr.	7:00 am/5 pm	584-2300	Harry Mellon	653-1301
	Rapposelli Construction	7:00 am/5 pm	555-4200	Joe Rapposelli	798-4491
	R. Tomasetti & Son	7:00 am/5 pm	584-3226	Ray Tomasetti	571-2630
	Graham Dewatering	7:00 am/5 pm	521-1964	Tom Graham	521-6000
Backhoe	Meadowood Water Dept.	8:00 am/6 pm	555-7100	Tom Holmbeck	597-0220
Bulldozer, front-end	Tidewater Utility Contr.	7:00 am/5 pm	584-2300	Harry Mellon	653-1301
loader, air compressor	Rapposelli Construction	7:00 am/5 pm	555-4200	Joe Rapposelli	798-4491
	Hayes & Friend Rental Co.	7:00 am/5 pm	564-1400	Peter Hayes	569-4171
Crane, rigging	Conestoga Rigging Co.	7:00 am/5 pm	644-0227	Herman Allen	798-1901
	DeLong Crane Rental	7:00 am/5 pm	644-2827	Dottie DeLong	644-0901
	Douglas Crane Service	7:00 am/6 pm	581-5751	Dick Douglas	263-1821
Electric generator, lighting	Meadowood Power & Light	8:00 am/5 pm	555-7300	Cal Frink	555-0221
lighting	Mullin Electric Co.	8:00 am/5 pm	584-5221	Charles Mullin	626-7830
	Dunham & Hume Electric	7:00 am/4:30 pm	454-4127	Jack Hume	454-4104
	Graham Dewatering	7:00 am/5 pm	521-1964	Tom Graham	521-6000

Figure 3-10. Community resource list.

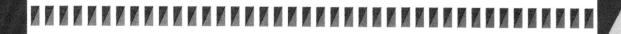

THE PARKWAY INCIDENT—
ASSESSMENT

We will zoom in on the rescue site now. Pop Edwards (the contractor) has met you and he has confirmed what the dispatcher has told you. You learn from him that there are no communication problems and that there are no injured persons outside the trench. You and he start toward the trench, and you begin your primary assessment. Note in the spaces below what you can perceive about hazards from the information on the site plan. The numbers indicate where you are when you make the observation.

1. Traffic? _____

2. Spectators? _____

3. Downed wires? _____

4. Well-point system? _____

5. Deep-well system? _____

6. Tripping hazards? _____

7. Disrupted utilities? _____

8. Flammable liquids? _____

9. Methane gas? _____

10. Exposed but unbroken utilities? _____

11. Flowing water? _____

Do you know how many people are completely buried? _____

Partially buried? _____

Do you know where the completely buried people are? _____

How do you know this? _____

What clues would you look for if you are not sure where a workmen is buried? _____

_____

Can you make the rescue with the people and equipment that you have on hand? Use the form (Figure 3-11) to assess your capabilities. Indicate by a checkmark in the first column what supplies and equipment you have carried to the scene. Then indicate with a checkmark in the second column what supplies and equipment you will require from community resources. Finally, indicate on the form how many rescuers and other emergency service personnel are likely to be on your first-responding units, and how many that you think you will need for the rescue operation. When you are finished, you should have a pretty good idea as to your first-response capabilities.

The emergency services dispatcher will have to know what you require from community resources. Indicate below what you will need in the way of services, supplies, and equipment. The dispatcher will then consult his resource list and initiate the calls for help.

EQUIPMENT CAPABILITY CHECKLIST

Equipment Carried	Community Resources	
_____	_____	Sheeting
_____	_____	Shoring
_____	_____	Chainsaw
_____	_____	Rescue saw
_____	_____	Circular saw
_____	_____	Sledge hammer 8#
_____	_____	Sledge hammer 3#
_____	_____	Claw hammers
_____	_____	Shovels
_____	_____	Entrenching tools
_____	_____	Plastic buckets
_____	_____	Wrecking bars 18"
_____	_____	Pinch bars 60"
_____	_____	Folding rules
_____	_____	Retracting tapes
_____	_____	Roll-up tapes
_____	_____	Tool kit
_____	_____	Nylon rope
_____	_____	Polypropylene rope
_____	_____	Tarpaulins
_____	_____	Safety can (5 gallon)
_____	_____	Safety can (2½ gallon)
_____	_____	Scabs
_____	_____	Wedges
_____	_____	Nails 16#DBL.H.D.
_____	_____	Carpenters aprons
_____	_____	Saw horses
_____	_____	Wire rope slings
_____	_____	Generators
_____	_____	Power cables
_____	_____	Distribution boxes
	_____	Floodlights
_____	_____	Tripod stands
_____	_____	Smoke ejector
	_____	Utility blower
_____	_____	Extension tube
_____	_____	Handlites

Figure 3-11. Parkway checklist.

Equipment Carried	Community Resources	
_____	_____	Submersible pump
_____	_____	Trash pump
_____	_____	Suction hose
_____	_____	Discharge hose
_____	_____	Clampstick
_____	_____	Lineman's gloves
_____	_____	Weighted throwing line
_____	_____	Traffic cones
_____	_____	Flares
_____	_____	Wall ladders
_____	_____	Extension ladders
_____	_____	S.C.B.A.
_____	_____	Supplied air systems
_____	_____	Safety harnesses
_____	_____	Hard hats
_____	_____	Leather gloves
_____	_____	Safety glasses
_____	_____	Reeves sleeve
_____	_____	Basket stretcher
_____	_____	Backboard
_____	_____	Trauma kit
_____	_____	Water cooler
_____	_____	High energy food/drink
_____	_____	Atmospheric monitors

Companies Responding:

Special Units Responding:

Community Resources Responding:

Manpower:

Figure 3-11. *Continued*

I will need these services: _____

_____

I will need these supplies and equipment: _____

_____

_____

Your next task will be to assign your personnel to hazard control and support operations.

Hazard Control

KNOWLEDGE OBJECTIVES

The rescuer should be able to—

☑ Define relevant words and phrases

☑ Summarize activities of the hazard control phase of a trench rescue operation

☑ List items of protective clothing that should be worn during a trench rescue operation

☑ Define the terms "general area" and "rescue area" as they relate to a trench rescue operation

☑ List at least two steps that rescuers need to take to make the general area safe

☑ List at least eight steps that rescuers need to take to make the rescue area safe

☑ List at least three operations that specialists need to undertake in an effort to make the rescue area safe

☑ Describe procedures for making a trench safe with conventional sheeting and shoring

☑ Describe procedures for making a trench safe with a trench box

☑ Describe procedures for making a trench safe with a precast concrete structure

☑ Describe procedures for making a trench safe with makeshift sheeting and shoring materials

SKILLS OBJECTIVES

The rescuer working as an individual or as part of a team should be able to—

☑ Manage the flow of traffic at the scene of a trench accident

☑ Manage the movement of spectators at the scene of a trench accident

☑ With the proper safety equipment, removed downed wires from the immediate rescue area

☑ Dewater a trench

☑ Keep contractor-installed dewatering systems operating

☑ Make the trench lip safe

☑ Ventilate a trench

☑ Support unbroken utility lines

☑ Remove tripping hazards

☑ Position a safety observer

☑ Make a trench safe with conventional sheeting and shoring materials

☑ Make a trench safe with substitute or makeshift sheeting and shoring materials

WORDS AND PHRASES YOU MAY BE SEEING FOR THE FIRST TIME

Air knife. A pneumatic tool used to cut away dirt with a high-velocity jet of air.

Angle of repose. The greatest angle above the horizontal plane at which loose material (such as soil) will lie without sliding.

Blockade. A barrier placed to halt the flow of vehicle traffic.

Clamp stick. A nonconducting lineman's tool essential to the safe movement of energized electric wires.

Confined area. Any space that lacks ventilation; usually the space is larger in area than the point of entry.

Danger zone. The area surrounding an accident site. The site of a danger zone is proportional to the severity of on-the-scene hazards.

Detour. A plan or procedure for routing traffic away from the scene of an accident.

Flotation. In this case, the distribution of weights and forces over an area of unstable ground.

Ground pads. Full sheets of $\frac{5}{8}$- or $\frac{3}{4}$-inch plywood placed next to the trench lip. Ground pads distribute weight and forces over their surface area and thus minimize the possibility of rescuers creating a secondary cave-in.

Lane control. A procedure for maintaining traffic flow around an accident site by funneling vehicles into fewer lanes.

Lineman's gloves. A set of nonconducting gum rubber gloves and protective leather shells used when it is necessary to work with a downed wire.

Mine drift. A nearly horizontal mine passageway.

Parallel trench. A previously excavated and back-filled trench close to and paralleling the trench being dug.

Perimeter. In this case, a real or imaginary line established around the accident site to direct the movement of spectators.

Replacement sewer line. A new pipeline installed next to an existing line for the purpose of taking over the original line's function.

Rescue area. Generally the area 50 feet in all directions from the accident site.

Sanitary sewer. A buried pipeline that carries sewage.

Select fill. Soil that is specially chosen to replace that which has been excavated.

Shotgun. Another term for a clamp stick, so named because of the slide action of the wire grip.

Storm sewer. A buried pipeline that carries surface water (such as rain water).

Sump. A pit dug at a low point in a trench floor; it serves to keep the screened end of a suction hose below the water level.

Tension cracks. Cracks in the ground adjacent to the trench. Tension cracks indicate that the ground has shifted; they should be considered warning signs.

Ventilating the trench. Using a powered fan to replace stale or contaminated air in a trench with fresh air.

Water table. The upper limit of a portion of the ground that is wholly saturated with water from underground sources. May be very near the surface or deep in the ground.

Weighted throwing line. One hundred feet of a nonconductive synthetic-fiber rope used for moving a downed wire when a clamp stick is not available. Steel rings or weighted wood blocks on the ends of the rope aid in achieving distance when the rope is thrown.

In the fourth phase of a rescue operation, rescuers must neutralize whatever hazards pose a threat to everyone who may be in or near the danger zone: the victims, workmen and spectators, other emergency service personnel, and, of course, the rescuers themselves. A wide variety of hazards may be found at the scene of a trench accident, including downed wires, broken utility lines in or near the trench, methane gas, and heavy equipment made unstable by the shifting ground. But the most severe danger is the one that rescuers often ignore: the trench itself!

The suggested hazard control steps are listed in a certain order. In a limited manpower–trench rescue operation, the steps might be carried out in that order. But when there are sufficient emergency service personnel at the accident site, hazard control operations may be carried out simultaneously.

SEEING THAT RESCUERS ARE PROTECTED

As a firefighter or rescuer, you have undoubtedly been conditioned to wear a full set of protective clothing in every emergency situation—including a helmet, eye protection, a turnout coat, gloves and boots, and perhaps even turnout pants. This gear and a breathing apparatus afford optimum protection against smoke and heat, falling objects, sharp objects, and other hazards common to a fire or accident scene.

In a trench rescue operation you may find that "regulation" protective gear is not particularly well suited for the activity, however. The front brim and neck protector of a standard firefighter's helmet may get in the way if you have to work in confined spaces. A regulation coat may not only be too warm when the temperature is high, but also too bulky. Even ordinary fire boots may pose a problem. If you become mired in the mud that is common to trench bottoms, you may find it extremely difficult to pull free.

Since there are usually no heat and sharp object hazards encountered in a trench rescue operation, I suggest that you consider the following items for your personal protection:

- **A construction-style helmet.** An ordinary "hard hat" offers excellent protection against falling objects (such as dirt and stones) without the extended brim and neck protector. If you have a helmet with a chin strap, remember to keep the strap fastened. A helmet that will not stay on is of little value.

- **Eye protection.** Spectacle-type glasses afford protection against flying particles of dirt that strike the face from the side or from below during digging operations in dry trenches.
- **Work clothes.** Ordinary work clothes are excellent for trench rescue operations. They should be close-fitting so that there is no chance for material to become trapped by dirt or stone. They should not be so snug that they impede movement when you are climbing over or under shoring devices or around dirt piles, however. Button the collar and the wrists to keep dirt out.
- **Gloves.** Close-fitting pigskin or goatskin gloves are well suited for shoring and digging operations.
- **Work shoes.** A pair of sturdy high-top work shoes with steel toes offers good foot protection. Also, these can be pulled more easily from mud.

Whatever you choose for protective gear, wear it! Always keep in mind that an injured rescuer is of no value to a rescue operation.

MAKING THE GENERAL AREA SAFE

You will see two terms used in the next few paragraphs: the "general" area and the "rescue" area. Let us consider the "general" area to be a space of indefinite size around the trench. It may be only a few hundred feet wide, or it may include several blocks. But within the area are cars, trucks, heavy machines, and people—all of which can be potentially dangerous to the rescue operation. The "rescue" area, as the term suggests, is the area close to the rescue site and usually extends for no more than a few dozen feet in any direction from the trench.

MANAGING TRAFFIC

The first effort in hazard control activities should be halting the flow of traffic over roads close to the accident site. Moving vehicles pose a threat to emergency service personnel working in the area. But the real danger is the severe vibrations caused by passing vehicles, especially heavy tractor-trailer combinations. Remember that these rigs can weigh as much as 80,000 pounds legally, and more with a permit.

Traffic control is generally the responsibility of police officers. However, if yours is the first emergency service unit on the scene, you may have to assign some of your personnel to traffic control duties, at least until police units arrive.

There are three basic traffic-management techniques: land control, blockading, and detouring. Do not consider lane control, even when it seems feasible to keep open at least one or two lanes of a super-highway. Vibrations can extend for a considerable distance when soil conditions are right. Detouring is the means of choice to keep traffic flowing, but it takes time to establish a detour. So when traffic poses a threat to the safety of victims and emergency service personnel, simply stop everything.

ESTABLISHING A BLOCKADE

Halting vehicles involves more than merely raising your hand and signaling the driver. This is especially true when vehicles are moving at high speeds. The driver of the nearest vehicle will probably be able to stop, but drivers behind him, unaware of the problem, may not.

Simply placing a string of traffic-warning devices along the side of the roadway may not be an effective way to stop vehicles on a high-speed road, either. When the road is heavily traveled it will not take long for the pavement adjacent to the markers to become filled. Nonetheless, some warning devices should be set out in such a manner that approaching drivers will see at least one or two of the markers before they realize that the vehicle ahead is stopped. Light sticks are a good substitute for flares.

DETOURING TRAFFIC

When traffic has been blockaded, a detour must be established so that vehicles will not clog the roadways that emergency units need to travel.

A detour should meet the following criteria:

- The alternate road should take traffic back to the primary route as quickly as possible.
- The detour should be able to accommodate the volume of traffic using the primary road; otherwise a blockade condition will continue to exist.
- There must be no bridges on the alternate route that are rated for less than the weight of the vehicles using the road.
- There must be no overpasses so low that the highest trucks using the alternate route cannot pass under them.
- There must be no hills that are too steep for heavy trucks that may have to use the road.
- The detour route must be clearly marked so that motorists unfamiliar with the area will not become lost.

If an alternate route meets these standards, an effective detour can be created.

Again, establishing a detour is usually a job for police officers, but when police officers are not available, the task may fall to fire and rescue personnel.

If it is your responsibility to establish a detour,

see that traffic flows to the right from the point of the blockade. Then there is no need for opposing traffic to be stopped while vehicles are channeled onto the detour route. Arrange warning devices so that drivers will have no trouble determining the direction in which they are to turn. When a detour starts at an intersection, direct traffic personally so that vehicles being detoured can be integrated into crossing traffic with a minimum of delay.

USING NON-EMERGENCY SERVICE PERSONNEL

There undoubtedly will be times when there are not enough rescuers and police officers on the scene to cope with traffic problems. In these cases you may have to rely on bystanders to keep traffic moving.

You should be wary of spectators who come forward to volunteer their services. Although they may have sound motives, these people may not have the slightest idea of what to do. Their efforts may only make the traffic problem worse. Instead, you should recruit such people as truck drivers and bus and taxi operators. These people make their living on the road, and they have probably experienced every sort of traffic situation. Accordingly, they usually have a knowledge of basic traffic-control measures.

When someone outside of the emergency services is recruited for traffic duty, he should be given clear and uncomplicated instructions. Leave nothing to chance! Your direction "Go down the road and put out some flares" could mean different things to different people. "Down the road" to one person might mean 15 feet; to another person it might mean 1500 feet, and in neither case would the flares be placed where you wanted them. To one person, "put out some flares" might mean the indiscriminate scattering of a few flares at the side of the road. Another person might think that you want him to stretch a line of flares completely across the highway.

Instead of being vague, leaving an order open to interpretation, you should say, "Go south on the road for 150 feet. Place one flare where the road meets the shoulder. As you walk back toward the rescue scene, place flares every 20 feet along the edge of the roadway." There should be very little question in a person's mind after he receives such an order.

> ### Remember
> Managing traffic should be the first hazard control activity. If traffic bogs down around the accident site, there not only will be a problem of getting emergency vehicles into the area. There will also be a problem in getting vehicles and people out of the area if other serious hazards—such as leaking gas and ruptured utility lines—are discovered. Initiating traffic control measures takes only a few minutes and those minutes are well spent when the rescue operation is complex and long-term.

MANAGING SPECTATORS

Spectators are drawn to a trench accident just as they are attracted to fires and vehicle accidents. As at fires and vehicle accidents, they can get in the way of emergency service personnel at trench accident scenes. Worse yet, they can cause a secondary collapse of trench walls if they are allowed to approach the edge of the trench. Crowd control must be an early consideration during hazard control efforts.

As your first step, set up a perimeter for spectators, preferably several hundred feet from the trench. It's important that you do this quickly, for once people congregate at an accident scene, they are usually reluctant to move. Follow this rule when establishing a perimeter for spectators: if they can see what is going on, they are too close!

Establishing a hypothetical perimeter (simply telling people to stay back) is a waste of time and effort. You must erect some sort of physical barrier, flimsy as it may be. Specially marked plastic perimeter tapes and high-visibility $\frac{3}{8}$-inch polypropylene ropes make excellent crowd control devices. Place them 3 to 4 feet above the ground.

If you are operating on city streets, have crowd control lines established at least a block away from the accident scene. This will be relatively easy since buildings, utility poles, and street signs are available for use as tie points.

Erecting perimeter lines may be more difficult in rural areas unless there are a number of trees and utility poles close to the site. However, the problem of finding suitable tie points can be solved by carrying with you a dozen or more 5-foot-long steel wire fence stakes. These are generally available in large hardware and farm equipment stores. They are ideal for the task; they are pointed and you can easily drive them into the ground by stepping on the tread plate. Place the stakes about 50 feet apart and secure the perimeter tape or the rope to the stakes.

When you deny access to a trench accident scene, deny access to everyone, including reporters, photographers, television crew members, and even emergency service personnel who are not directly concerned with the rescue effort. Never lose sight of the fact that the weight of even one nonessential person can cause a secondary cave-in. Once the trench is made safe, the news media can be handled by your public relations officer. Procedures for dealing with the news media are discussed in Phase 5—Support Operations.

Like traffic control, crowd control should be a function of police officers. But when police personnel are not immediately available, you should be prepared for the task.

MAKING THE RESCUE AREA SAFE

With traffic halted or diverted and spectators kept at a safe distance, you can attend to the hazards that may be present within the rescue area. Keep in mind that there may be not only more hazards, but also vastly different kinds of hazards from those encountered at fire and vehicle accident scenes. Some of these hazards can be neutralized by rescue personnel; some can be made ineffective only by specialists.

CONTROLLING HAZARDS CREATED BY DISRUPTED UTILITIES

The utility hazards produced by a trench accident that you can control (if you have the equipment) are downed wires, replacement sewer lines, and broken water service lines.

DOWNED WIRES

Imagine the possibility of a nearby utility pole becoming dislodged when a trench wall gives way. The pole may remain supported by the wires, but it may fall and carry broken wires to the area close to the trench.

You will not have to wait for personnel from the utility company to reach the scene if your unit is equipped with a pair of lineman's gloves and a lineman's clamp stick (often called a "shotgun") or a special weighted throwing line. Follow this procedure:

First, quickly field-test the rubber gloves. Stretch the cuff edges between your fingers and, while holding them tightly, twirl the glove so that air is trapped inside. Hold each inflated glove close to your face so that you can listen and feel for leaks from pinholes, which make the gloves unsafe. If the test is satisfactory, put on the gloves and the leather protective shells.

If you have a clamp stick, approach the wire from the broken end, if possible so that the wire cannot touch you if it arcs and whips. Grip the wire about 12 to 18 inches from its end. Keep the clamp stick between you and the wire so that "reel curl" will cause the wire to move away from you if it detaches from the clamp stick. Move the wire to a safe place with the clamp stick and hold it to the ground while another squadman weights it down with a piece of wood, a coil of rope, or some other object. Post a guard near the wire to warn people away from the danger.

A weighted throwing line can be made with a 100-foot-length of synthetic fiber rope (preferably polydacron) and two steel rings or other reasonably heavy objects. Manila fiber rope should never be used for moving downed wires.

Put on the lineman's gloves and shells and take up a position at the side of the wire. Loosely coil half of the rope in your hand while you stand on the midpoint (usually marked in some way). Throw one weighted end under the wire and the other weighted end over the wire. Move to where the weighted ends have landed, pick them up, and drag the wire to a safe place. The 50 feet of rope will create a safe distance between you and the wire. Have someone weight the wire and post a guard.

It is important to realize that this is not all the information you need to move a downed wire. You should know something about conductivity, the effect of electricity, ground effect, and other vital factors. This knowledge can be gained only by attending a formal training program directed by an expert.

REPLACEMENT SEWER LINES

You may arrive on the scene of a trench accident and find that raw sewage is pouring into the open trench. The contractor was probably installing a replacement line and did not plug the old pipe. In this situation, a trapped workman can quickly drown. You must initiate dewatering operations immediately.

A trash pump is ideal for this task if you can find one on the job site. If a trash pump is not available, use the submersible electric pump or the gasoline-powered pump from your rig. Either of these pumps will be able to move the liquid portion of the sewage if the inlet is fitted with a strainer.

Drop the submersible pump or the hard sleeve of the portable pump into the trench at a low point and begin pumping. Do not pump raw sewage into the street. Instead, have squadmen extend the discharge line to the next downhill manhole. Remember that most sewers are laid uphill, so you can generally find the next downhill manhole by looking past the trench end opposite the backhoe.

BROKEN WATER SERVICE LINES

Water service lines are pipes that branch off of street mains and supply adjacent buildings. If a water service line has been broken by the trench collapse and water is flowing into the trench, you will either have to devise a way to shut off the flow or wait for water department personnel to arrive. You may be able to stop, or at least slow, the flow by closing the end of the pipe between two hammers, or perhaps by squeezing the pipe shut with a hydraulic tool. A cooper line can generally be crimped shut without difficulty.

> **Remember**
> The three hazard control measures just described cannot be accomplished in a totally safe environment. You will have to work near or even over the edge of the trench. Stay as far from the lip as you can, but when you have to work near, do so while wearing a full body harness with a rope held by two other rescuers in a safe area. In any event, never enter an unshored trench. Ground pads, such as those described under "Making the Trench Lip Safe," should be used immediately.

HAVING SPECIALISTS CONTROL SPECIAL HAZARDS

It will not be possible for you to control all of the hazards that may be encountered at the scene of a trench accident. It will be necessary for you to call upon a variety of community resource personnel for assistance before you can make the trench safe and initiate the actual rescue effort. Remember, "Thou Shalt Not Fry Thy Help!"

BROKEN GAS MAINS

If during your assessment you discover a broken gas main, you should not attempt a rescue. You should evacuate the area for a considerable distance and stand by until the gas company can shut off the flow. A high-order explosion may be imminent, especially if there are sources of ignition nearby.

You should be aware that open flames and sparks are not the only sources of ignition for natural gas in a trench. Static electricity can also ignite gas and can be generated in the very pipe that is carrying the flammable gas.

DISRUPTED UNDERGROUND ELECTRICAL CONDUITS

Buried conduits often carry high-voltage, high-amperage electricity. If you see that such a conduit has been broken during a trench collapse, immediately notify the power company and stand by until the circuit is disconnected.

BROKEN WATER MAINS

Water can flow through mains at the rate of a few hundred to several thousand gallons per minute, depending on the size of the main and the water pressure. Water flowing from a broken main poses a dual threat. It can, of course, drown trapped victims. It also can contribute to the secondary collapse of trench walls.

While you are waiting for water department personnel to shut off the flow, set up pumps and commence dewatering operations. Be sure that pumps are not placed so close to the edge of the trench that they will cause its collapse. You may eventually have to dig a sump so that the water level can be lowered beyond the digging area. However, this should not be done until the remaining trench walls are made safe with sheeting and shoring or some other means.

RUPTURED STEAM, CHEMICAL, AND FUEL LINES

Contractors working in or near industrial plants often uncover steam, chemical, and fuel lines, either by accident or design. If they know such lines exist, they can take special care not to break them during the excavation operations. It is when no one knows of these lines that they are broken during digging. If you are confronted with a broken high-pressure steam line, chemical line, or fuel line, quickly call for help from the plant in which the line originates or terminates. Stand by until the hazard is controlled.

KEEPING DEWATERING SYSTEMS OPERATING

When a trench is dug near a body of water, or in ground that is saturated because of a high water table, contractors install deep wells or well-point systems. The pumps that are connected to the systems continually draw water which can seep into the trench and fill it, from the ground.

If there is a well-point system operating at the site of a trench accident, it is vitally important that you keep the system operating. If necessary, post a guard to see that no workmen, rescuers, or spectators inadvertently shut the system down.

Anytime you observe either ground or surface water in a trench, your mental "red flag" should go up. Start thinking in terms of increasing the size of wales, and perhaps shoring.

MAKING THE TRENCH LIP SAFE

Once hazards have been controlled by rescuers or community resource personnel, you can turn your attention to making the trench lip safe. If a number of rescuers have to walk near the lip of the trench, their combined weights may result in downward forces that are sufficient to cause the trench wall to collapse. But if the weight of the rescuers is spread over a wide area, the downward forces are minimized and the chance of a secondary cave-in is lessened.

Lay down ground pads (4- by 8-foot sheets of $\frac{5}{8}$- or $\frac{3}{4}$-inch plywood) parallel to the side of the trench opposite the spoil pile. There will probably be no room for these pads on the side of the spoil pile. If there is not, lay down 2- by 12-inch planks. It may be necessary to clear a space between the edge

of the trench and the pile; do this carefully with a shovel.

For assessment, approach the trench from the end (the narrowest side). Do not go closer than 4 feet. This is close enough for observation. Next, level the ground between the trench and the spoil pile to accept the 2- by 12-inch planks that will serve as ground pads. Stand on a two-by-twelve as you level the ground, then slide the plank forward. Do this every 3 feet. Be aware that you may have to move a large quantity of dirt because the contractor may have piled the spoil right next to the trench (even though the law specifically requires that it be a minimum of 2 feet from the trench lip). There is no need to dig down to the original ground; simply level off where it is convenient. Refer to Figures 4-1, 4-2, and 4-3.

Next, place the 4- by 8-foot panels as ground pads along the trench, opposite the spoil pile. It is good to start with the end panel across the end of the trench, and then place the panels all the way along the length of the trench that encompasses the work area. Overlap the panels by 6 inches as you place them and make sure that they extend to the very edge of the lip (Figures 4-4 and 4-5).

If for any reason the spoil pile has to be moved (such as if the spoil is piled up on both sides of the trench, thus compounding the danger to the rescuers), place a large backhoe (in excess of 1 yard) on the back side of the spoil pile and drag the dirt back. Certainly, if they are available, a backhoe on each side will be much faster.

The engines of these backhoes will not cause too much vibration. **Do *not* use either cat-mounted or rubber-tired front-end loaders or bulldozers to do this job.** The vibratory results could be disastrous. You want to avoid the actual movement of machinery.

Keep in mind that by laying down ground pads you may be covering tension cracks that appear as a warning of unstable ground. It may seem dangerous to cover these cracks; however, the flotation feature of pads far outweighs the desirability of leaving the cracks exposed. You already know that you have a soil stability problem.

POSITIONING A SAFETY OBSERVER

Position a rescuer at one end of the trench throughout the sheeting and shoring operations. Have him watch for cracks and pieces of falling dirt and stone—signs of an impending secondary wall collapse. This person will serve as the "Competent Person." As described by OSHA, a competent person is "one who is capable of identifying existing and predicable hazards in the surrounding or working conditions which are unsanitary, hazardous, or dangerous to employees and who has authorization

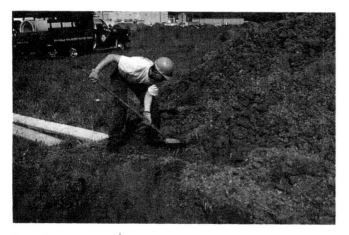

Figure 4-1. Level ground for ground planks.

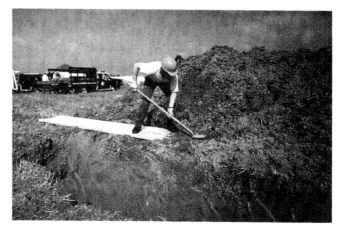

Figure 4-3. Continue this action until plank is in position.

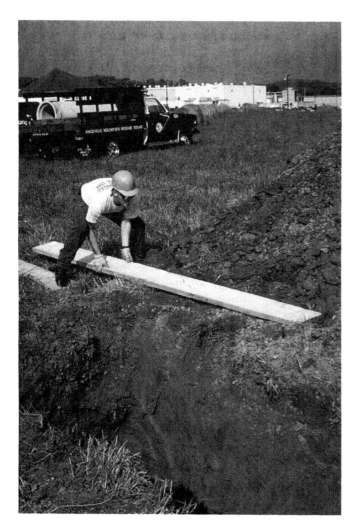

Figure 4-2. Slide the plank forward every 3 feet.

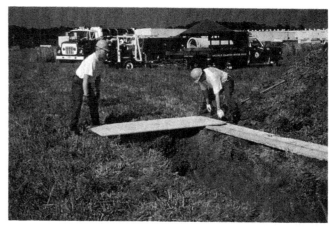

Figure 4-4. Place a ground panel across the end of the trench.

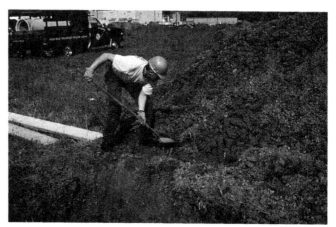

Figure 4-5. Overlap planks and panels 6 inches.

to take prompt corrective measures to eliminate them."

The safety observer, or "competent person," should be given the job of monitoring the atmosphere in the trench, periodically using an appropri-

ate analyzer. He also will be responsible for making sure that the crew is properly dressed, and for the upkeep of the accountability time in–time out board. He will report to the trench boss as a second set of eyes.

MONITORING AND VENTILATING THE TRENCH

Once ground pads are down, rescuers can begin other operations to make the trench safe.

First, test the atmosphere in the trench by lowering an atmospheric monitor. Test the top, middle, and bottom of the trench as you would a confined space. Follow the manufacturer's instructions for your specific monitor. Test for oxygen content, hydrocarbons, and toxic gases in that order. Keep in mind that you are not only looking for methane, but also carbon monoxide and—the worst possibility—hydrogen sulphide. A large concentration of any of these gases may require the use of a breathing apparatus.

It is important to bear in mind that there are detectors that, when properly calibrated and operated, measure the concentration of all gases. Often gas detectors are purchased, played with for a short time, and then put into a compartment and never used until the time of an emergency. Rescuers must practice with gas detectors if they are to become proficient with them.

If you find that there is a dangerous concentration of gas in the air, you have to ventilate the trench. It is best, then, to adopt the practice of ventilating all trenches, first determining the presence, kind, and severity of the gas. You need to establish these criteria to give yourself something to base future tests on. The trench may have been dug in ground that is directly over a landfill, in ground that has been used to fill a marsh, or in ground that covers a mine drift. In any of these or other cases, methane gas may be seeping through the ground into the trench.

To effectively ventilate a trench, place a fresh-air blower or a smoke ejector so that air directed into the excavation sweeps out the dangerous gases. The blower or fan should be capable of moving a minimum 1000 cubic feet of air per minute.

Polypro pipe is widely used throughout the country for the transmission of natural gas. If you find that polypro pipe is being used as the conductor of natural gas, not only must you ventilate the trench, you must also provide a means for draining off static electricity that may cause the ignition of methane.

Studies have shown that the ignition of natural gas can result from static electricity when—

- There is sufficient gas flow in the pipe to cause extreme turbulence.
- There are rust particles or other foreign particles in the pipe.
- The static charge is present at a point along the pipe where there is an ideal mixture of gas and air.

You can minimize the possibility of a gas explosion by draining the static charge from the pipe. The procedure is simple: Wipe the exposed section of pipe with a wet cloth. Then drape the wet cloth over the plastic pipe so that the cloth touches the ground. You must keep the cloth wet; it will conduct the static charge from the pipe to the ground. **Never touch the exposed pipe with either your hand or a tool.**

Remember that only an exposed pipe can be drained of a static charge in this manner. If a secondary cave-in causes pipe to be exposed a short distance from the pipe that was exposed in the original cave-in, that section of pipe must be treated in the same way.

SUPPORTING UNBROKEN UTILITY LINES

Underground utility and supply lines may be purposely or accidentally uncovered during trench excavation operations. These lines may be parallel to the trench, or at a 90-degree angle to the excavation. Regardless of what an exposed pipe or conduit is carrying, it should be supported before the shoring and digging operations are begun, if possible.

Supporting unbroken utility lines can be accomplished in one of two ways (Figure 4-6). You can either lay a ladder across the trench and support the pipe with straps or ropes, or you can brace the pipe from below. The latter technique should be attempted only after the walls of the trench are made safe with sheeting and shoring, however. In either case, do not move the line in any direction; simply stabilize it.

An exposed utility line may be a valuable clue as to the condition of surrounding ground. Whenever you see an exposed pipe, whether it is parallel to the trench or at right angles, you should realize right away that you are not dealing with virgin

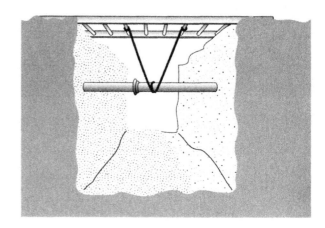

Figure 4-6. Supporting unbroken utilities.

ground. You are in an area where a parallel or bisecting trench has been dug before. You should also realize that because of this, the trench walls may be quite unstable. The following story will show how a trench-digging operation can be marked for disaster many years in advance.

In 1969, Contractor A was hired to install an 8-inch sanitary sewer line 8 feet deep in the center of Main Street. The material excavated was heavy red clay; however, the job specifications stated that the excavated clay was not suitable for backfill. The reason for this is that clay will not compact solidly; therefore it makes an unsuitable base for a new road. Thus the contractor was required to haul in "select fill"—in this case, sand that could be tightly compacted. Even though the resulting job was labeled "good and tight," the sand and clay would never become cohesive, or "stuck together."

In 1980, Main Street was very different. It had a new high school and many new commercial buildings. The old 8-inch sewer line was described as woefully inadequate, so the town fathers decided to have installed a new 15-inch sanitary sewer line 9 feet in the ground and 6 feet from the old line.

Contractor B opened a new trench 4 feet wide and 10 feet deep. Since he was digging in clay, he decided to take a chance and work without sheeting and shoring. When the trench was opened, there was only a 3-foot wall of clay between the new trench and the sandfill of the old trench, and the clay was not knit to the sand.

Consequently, the wall collapsed and the rescue squad was called to extricate trapped workmen. Both common sense and federal law dictated that the trench walls be made safe, but sheeting and shoring cost money, and—well you know the rest of the story.

REMOVING TRIPPING HAZARDS

Have rescuers remove batter boards, string lines, planks, tools, pipes, and anything else that might cause rescuers to trip and fall.

MAKING THE TRENCH SAFE

Using makeshift materials, or materials that do not meet standards required under the provisions of OSHA are not recommended.

USING APPROVED MATERIALS

So that emergency service personnel can work in as close to absolute safety as possible, shoring devices should be even stronger than those required by OSHA and placement patterns should exceed those mandated in the charts. For example:

- All uprights shall be at least 2- by 12-inch planks.
- Maximum spacing of shores (crossbraces) shall be 4 feet both horizontally and vertically.
- The minimum number of horizontal shores or crossbraces, whether timbers, screw jacks, or pneumatic, required for each pair of uprights shall be determined by the number of 4-foot zones into which the depth of the trench may be divided. One horizontal shore shall be required for each of these zones, but in no case shall there be less than two shores. Trenches in which depth cannot be divided into these standard zones shall have an extra horizontal shore supplied for the short remaining zone, if the zone is greater than half the 4-foot zone.
- A sheeting and shoring operation shall not be used for trenches deeper than 15 feet.

TYPES OF TRENCH ACCIDENTS

There are many types of trench accidents. Space limitations prohibit discussion of techniques for making trenches safe for every possible situation; the combinations of situations and hazard control measures are just too numerous. Accordingly, we will consider techniques for making trenches safe in those situations that are most likely to occur: when the spoil pile slides, when a side wall shears, where there is a slough-in, when one side of the trench caves in, and when both sides of the trench cave in. Sheeting and shoring "T" trenches, "X" trenches, "L" trenches, and hand-dug shallow wells will be explained.

In the illustrations that follow, the trench in which the rescuers are shown working is 4 feet wide by about 30 feet long, with the affected section about 8 feet long—an "average" trench. Needless to say, you will have to use longer shores when it is necessary to make a wider trench safe, and additional sheeting when a larger portion of the trench is affected by the soil movement.

SPOIL-PILE SLIDES/SIDE-WALL SHEARS/SLOUGH-INS

Spoil-pile slides, side-wall shears, and slough-ins are grouped together because the same technique for making the trench safe can be used in any of the three. So that you can better understand what happens in each situation, refer to the next three illustrations.

Figure 4-7 illustrates a spoil-pile slide. This usually results when the backhoe operator piles the excavated earth too close to the trench lip and at too steep an angle. The soil slides into the trench.

Figure 4-8 illustrates a side-wall shear. A portion of the wall simply shears away and falls into the trench. This is a common occurrence in clay and wet sand.

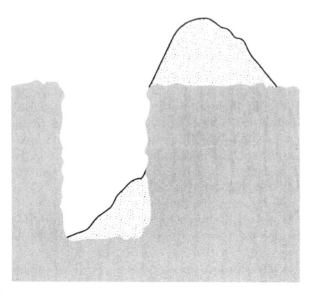

Figure 4-7. Spoil-pile slide.

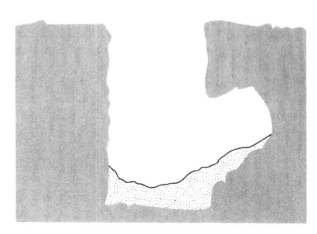

Figure 4-9. Slough-in.

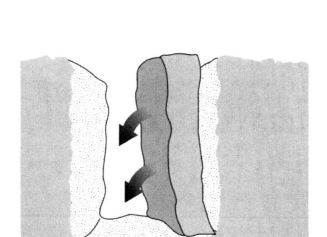

Figure 4-8. Side-wall shear.

Figure 4-9 illustrates a slough-in. In this case a portion of the side wall becomes detached and slides into the trench, leaving an overhang. This type of movement is common in wet sand, clay, and a sand and gravel mix.

Note that in each of these situations the trench walls remain nearly vertical and serve as support for the sheeting.

A word of caution should be given here about slough-in–type accidents. The portion that becomes detached may be only a few inches thick; however, it can be several feet thick depending on soil conditions. **As a matter of safe practice, you should never attempt to sheet and shore a trench in which the slough-in is deeper than 18 inches.** Medium- and low-pressure air bags can be used successfully to fill in these voids between the sheeting and trench wall, although they may not be effective in every case. Stuff the bag(s) in the void behind the sheeting. Inflate until the bag is tight against the sheeting and shut off the air supply. Caution: overinflation will cause a blow-out of the sheeting.

Let us discuss how a trench can be made safe with sheeting and timber shores.

USING SHEETING AND TIMBER SHORES

Be extremely careful to select proper-sized timber for shores. When the trench is less than 10 feet deep and 6 feet wide, use 4- by 4-inch timbers for shores. When the trench is from 6 to 9 feet wide and less than 10 feet deep, use 4- by 6-inch timbers for shores. The size of timbers selected for shores is always relevant to the depth and width of the trench.

Even though the trench may be only 8 feet deep, start with three shores on the first set of panels as a safety precaution and for ease of installation. From then on, follow the rule of one shore for each 4-foot zone.

Some steps that were discussed earlier in this phase will be repeated in an effort to maintain continuity. Among them will be such steps as making the trench lip safe and ventilating and monitoring the atmosphere in the trench.

We will make these assumptions: the area around the trench has been cleared, and equipment to be used for the rescue operation has been placed near the trench.

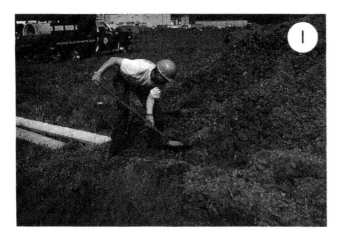

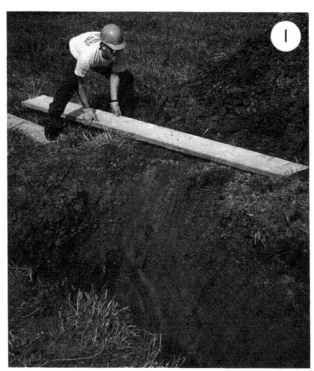

Step 1. Level the ground between the edge of the trench and the body of the spoil pile and lay down 2- by 12-inch planks. These planks will serve as ground pads. ▲ ▶

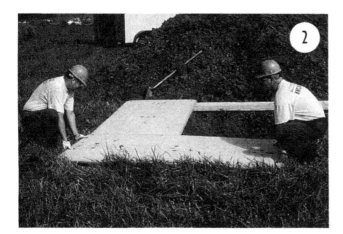

Step 2. Lay down 4- by 8-foot panels adjacent to the trench lip on the side of the trench opposite the spoil pile. These panels should be placed end to end so that there is a continuous walkway and should extend for several feet on each side of the affected area. ▲

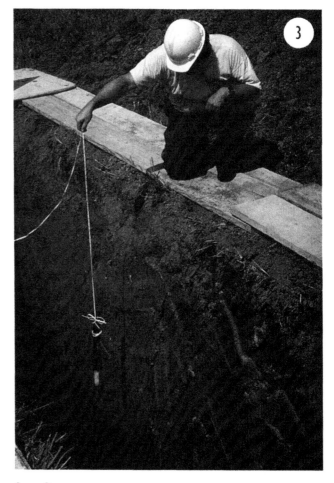

Step 3. Monitor the atmospheric conditions in the trench. ▲

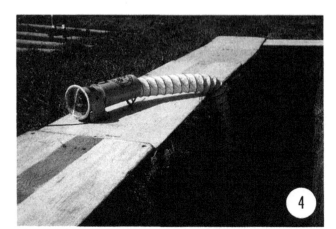

Step 4. Ventilate the trench.

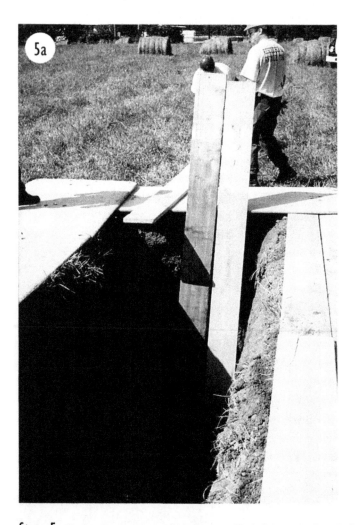

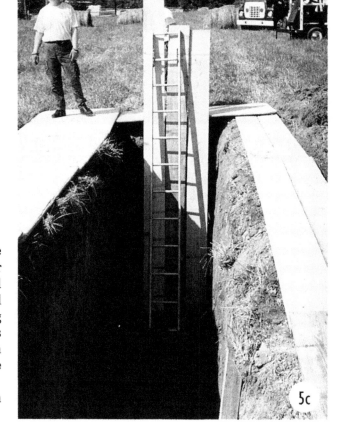

Step 5. It is time to "safe" the end of the trench. If the trench is wider than 4 feet, you must treat it as a face or wall by installing a panel. Run the shores on a diagonal into the sides of the uprights, both on the end panel and the trench panels. Do not align the shores with existing shores. Toe-in the shores with nails. If the trench is less than 4 feet wide, we can simply lay 2-inch by 12-inch by 12-foot planks vertically at a slight angle into the trench. Any breakaway of soil or clumps of soil will fall harmlessly, straight down. The planks will keep them from bouncing out into the trench. ▲ ▶ ◀

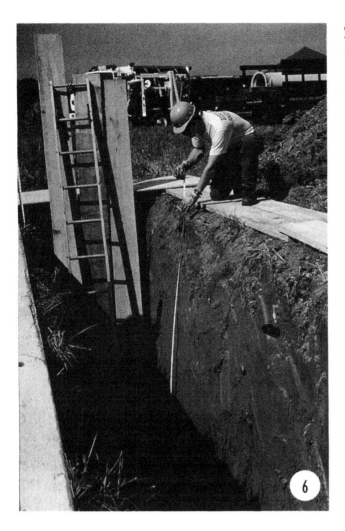

Step 6. Measure the depth of the trench on one side. ◀

Note

Two measurements are necessary since the floor of the trench may be quite uneven. For the sake of clarity, we will consider here that the floor of the trench is practically level. Figures 4-11 through 4-14 will illustrate what to do when the floor is uneven.

Step 7. Measure the depth of the trench on the other side. ▶

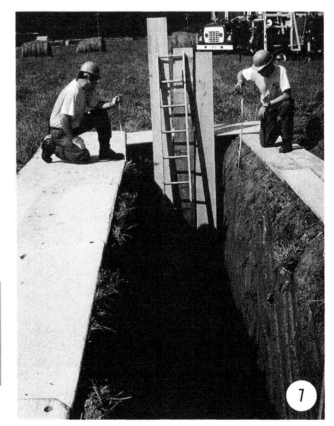

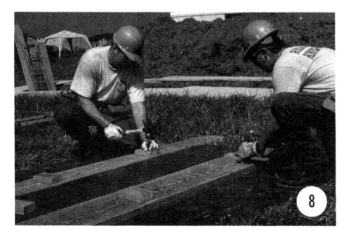

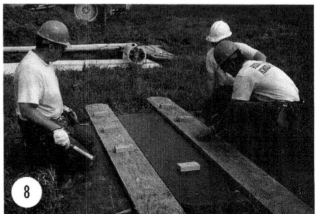

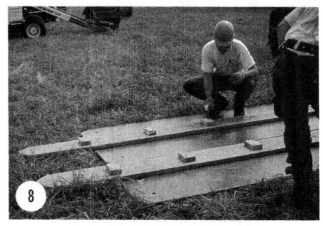

Step 8. Place the prefabricated panels side by side and even, since the floor of the trench is level. Nail the scabs that will support the shores. Secure each scab with two nails. Position the scabs so that the shores will be evenly spaced throughout the depth of the trench, but in no case position the scabs so that shores will be more than 4 feet apart. ▲ ▶ ▼

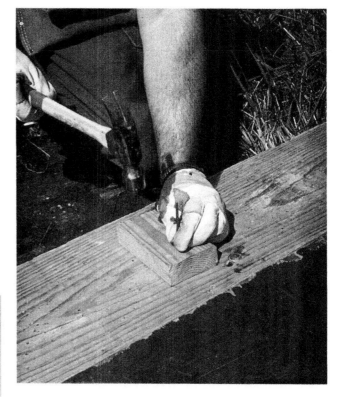

Note
To prevent the 2- by 4-inch scabs from splitting as they are nailed, blunt the point of each nail before driving it. Simply hold the nail head down on a firm surface and strike the point with the hammer face (Figure 4-10).

Figure 4-10. Blunt the sharp point to prevent splitting the scabs.

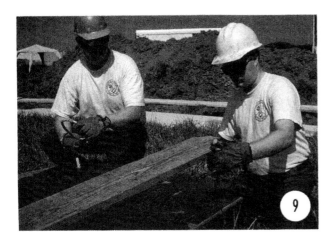

Step 9. Secure ropes to the panels. Use the holes if holes are provided. If the panels do not have holes, secure a single rope to the upright with a loop knot.
◄

Step 10. Turn one panel over and lower it into the trench with the upright facing in. ►

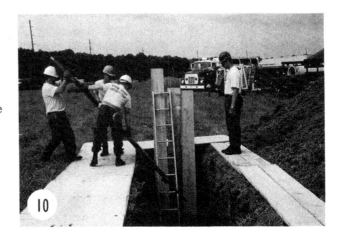

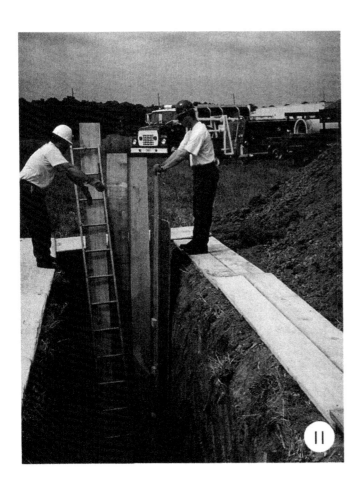

◄
Step 11. Pass the ropes to rescuers on the opposite side of the trench. Adjust the panel so that it stands vertically against the trench wall.

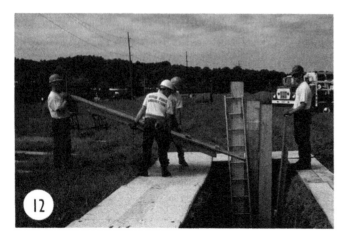

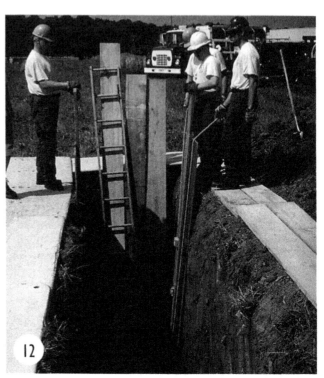

Step 12. While one rescuer holds the first panel in place, lower the second panel into the trench with the upright facing in. Make sure that the panels are directly opposite each other, and that each panel is snug against the trench wall and vertical. Two rescuers should continue to hold the panels vertically against the trench walls during the shoring operation. Thus they will be able to prevent the panels from slipping sideways. ▲ ▶

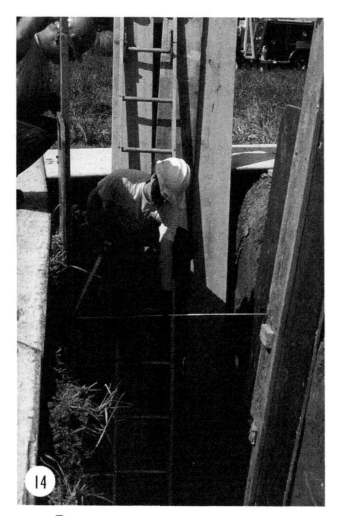

Step 13. Make sure that the ladder is close to the working area so that the rescuer installing the first shore will not have to reach over an unsafe distance.

Step 14. Climb down the ladder, but no deeper into the trench than waist-level. This will minimize the possibility of being completely buried in the event of a secondary cave-in. Measure the distance between the uprights at the top set of scabs. ◀

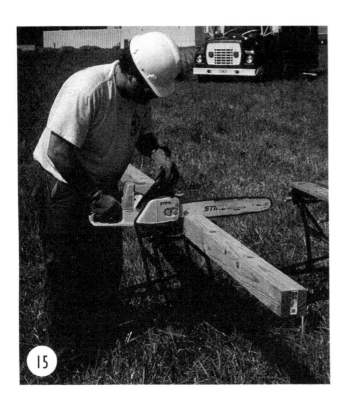

Step 15. Cut a piece of timber the appropriate length for the first shore.
◄

Step 16. Place the shore on the top set of scabs. It is important that you shore from the top down when using timbers. When the top shore is in place, there will be little chance for a secondary wall collapse or additional spoil-pile movement. ▶

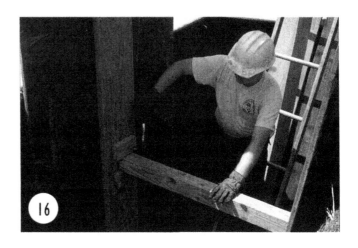

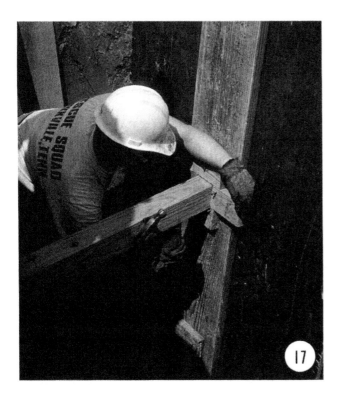

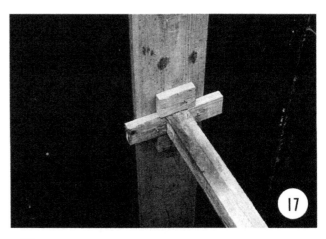

Step 17. Secure one end of the shore to the upright by nailing scabs around the other three sides of the shore. In other words, box the shore.
◄ ▲

Step 18. Measure and cut the center shore and position it on the scabs. If the shore is loose between the uprights, drive two wedges between the upright and the unboxed end of the shore. Use two short sledgehammers simultaneously so that the wedges are driven in uniformly. Do not drive the wedges so tight that they cause the bottom of the prefab panel to curve out. ▶

Step 19. Secure the wedges in place with a scab nailed to the upright. The ends of the wedges are left unsecured so that they can be used to tighten the shore later in the operation, if necessary.

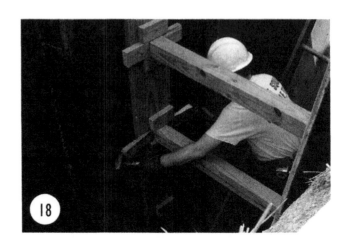

Step 20. Climb down the ladder and measure for the third shore.
◀

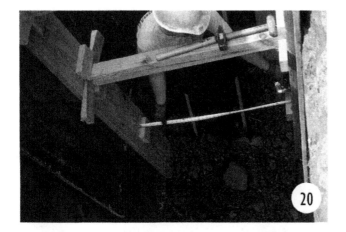

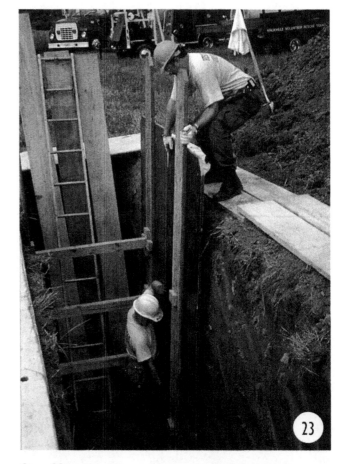

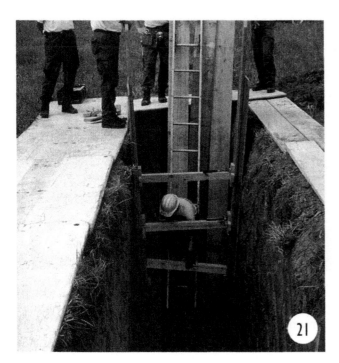

Step 21. Cut the third shore to the correct length. ▲

Step 22. Secure the bottom shore with scabs in the same way as the top and middle shores.

Step 23. Place a third panel against the spoil-pile side of the trench with the upright facing in. Be sure that the edge of this panel butts against the edge of the panel previously placed. ▲

Step 24. The rescuer in the trench can assist with the positioning of the next pair of panels since he can work out of the "safed" area.

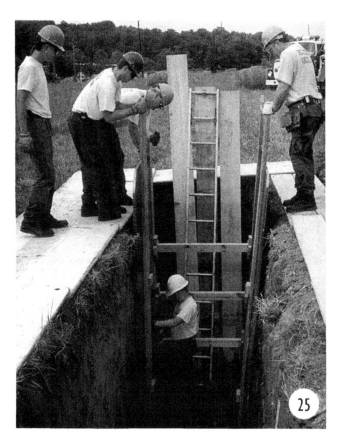

Step 25. Place the fourth panel in the trench with the upright facing in. Again, be sure that the edges of the panels butt against each other. Two rescuers should continue to hold the second set of panels so that they remain vertical during the shoring operation. ◀

Step 26. Measure for the bottom shore for the second set of panels. This departure from the procedure suggested for the first set of panels is possible because the rescuer can work out of the "safed" area. Note that the trench is 8 feet deep, thus we need only two shores per set of panels (two 4-foot zones).

Step 27. Place and secure the bottom and top shores, in that order. Box them in place and use wedges whenever the shores are loose between the uprights.

Step 28. Position a third set of panels. ◀

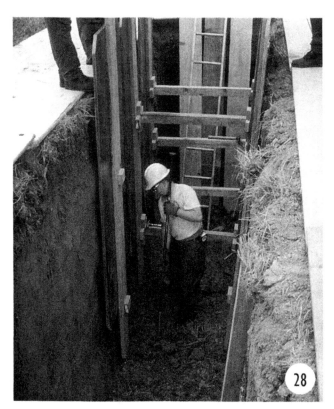

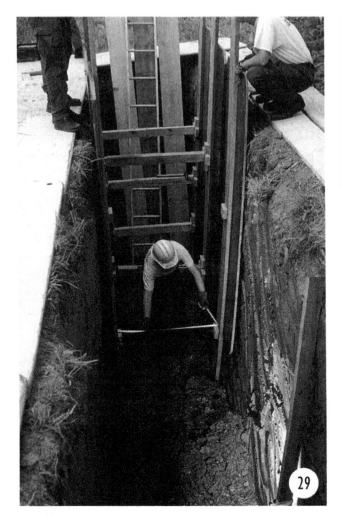

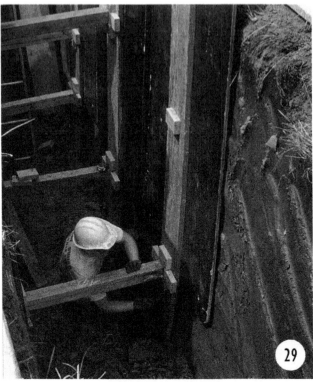

Step 29. Measure for and install shores in the same way as the first and second set of panels. ◀ ▲

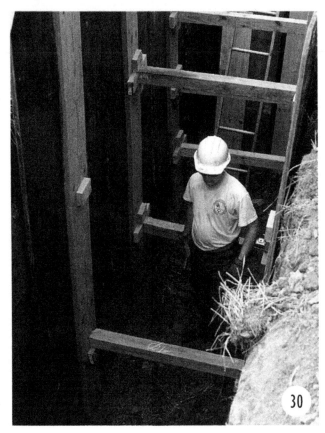

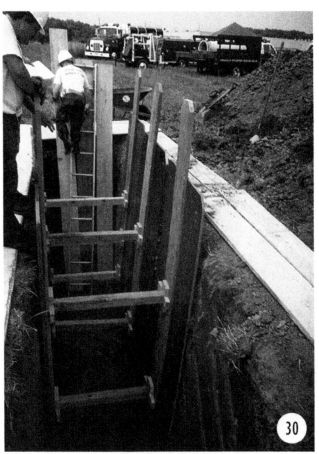

Step 30. Work from the bottom to the top and make sure that all scabs are nailed, as shown. ◀ ▲

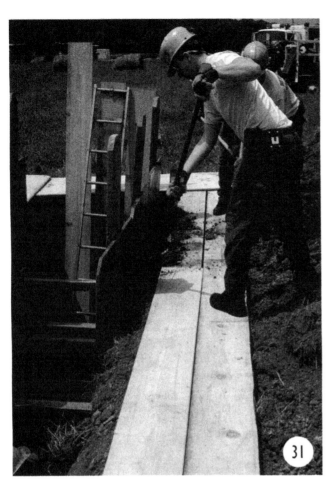

Step 31. Once the sheeting and shoring is installed, fill in any voids between the sheeting and trench wall with dirt from the spoil pile. This will lessen the chances for soil to move forcefully against the sheeting if there is additional earth movement. Warn rescuers in the trench before filling voids. The sound of earth moving against the sheeting can be rather unsettling to anyone in the trench! ◀

Step 32. Remove any debris that may have accumulated in the trench and prepare the trench floor for digging operations. ▶

Step 33. Make sure that the blower continues to operate during the sheeting, shoring, and digging operations.

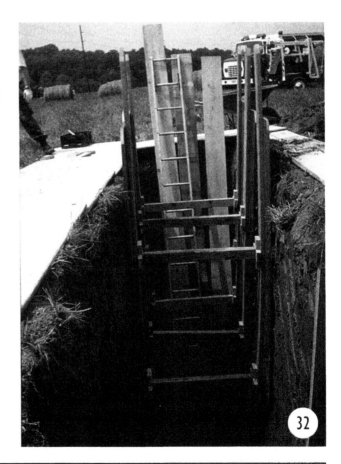

Before we go on to discuss the technique of shoring with screw jacks, consider the problem of an uneven trench floor.

Figure 4-11 shows a trench with a floor made uneven by a spoil-pile slide. By measuring each side, the rescuer will be able to determine just how much higher the panels of one side will be when they are positioned in the trench.

Figure 4-12 shows how the panels are laid out before the scabs are nailed in place. The panels are laid side by side, but one panel is offset for the difference that was determined by measuring both sides of the trench.

In Figure 4-13 you can see that the scabs of one panel are kept in line with those of the other panel as they are nailed.

When the panels are positioned in the trench, the shores will be horizontal, as you can see in Figure 4-14.

USING SHEETING AND SCREW JACKS

Speed can be added to a sheeting and shoring operation when screw jacks are used instead of timbers. There is no need for the boxing and wedging operations that are part of shoring with timbers, and measurements need not be as exact as when they are made for wood shores.

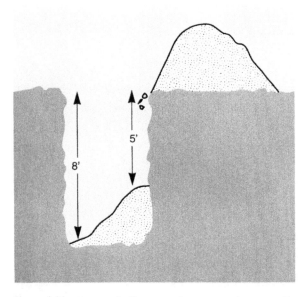

Figure 4-11. A trench floor made uneven by a spoil-pile slide.

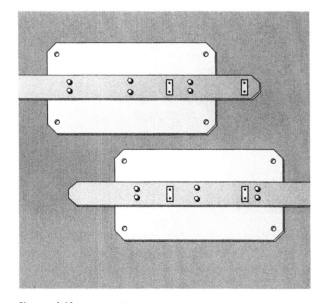

Figure 4-13. Keep the scabs on each panel in line with each other as they are nailed.

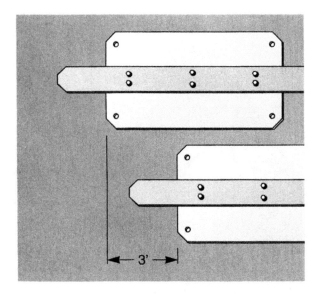

Figure 4-12. Lay out the panels side by side, offsetting one according to the measurement of the trench floor.

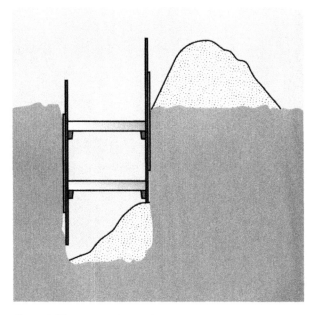

Figure 4-14. Correctly positioned panels.

You should be aware of these points when using screw jacks for shoring:

- Screw jacks and pipes should not be used for spans greater than 5 feet; long lengths of pipe tend to bend when there is considerable force exerted against the shoring.
- There are two different sizes of screw jacks. The smaller jacks should never be used with 2-inch pipe.

You may find this suggestion helpful if you choose to use screw jacks for a trench rescue operation: If you must use the combination of a socket butt and screw end for each shore instead of two screw ends, tape the socket-butt end to the pipe before lowering the shore into the trench (see Figure 4-15). When it is taped in place in this manner, the socket butt will not slip from the pipe as the shore is lowered into place. Figure 4-16 shows a typical installation.

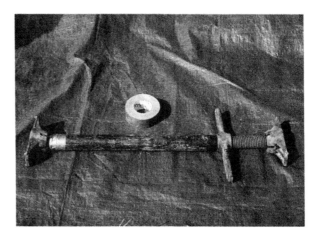

Figure 4-16. A typical installation.

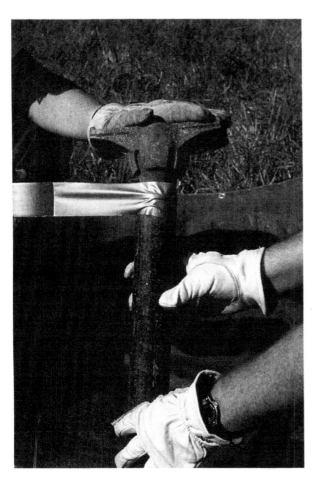

Figure 4-15. Tape the socket butt end to the pipe.

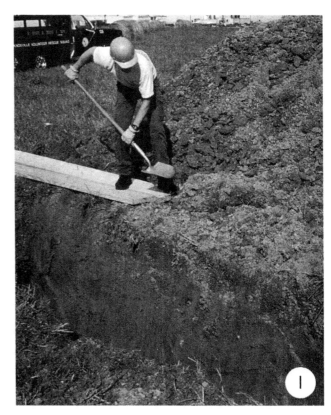

Step 1. Level the ground between the edge of the trench and the body of the spoil pile and lay down 2- by 12-inch planks. These planks will serve as ground pads. ▶

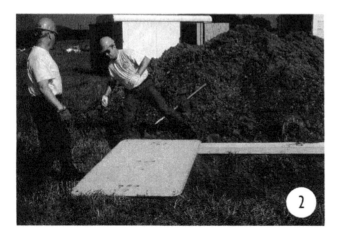

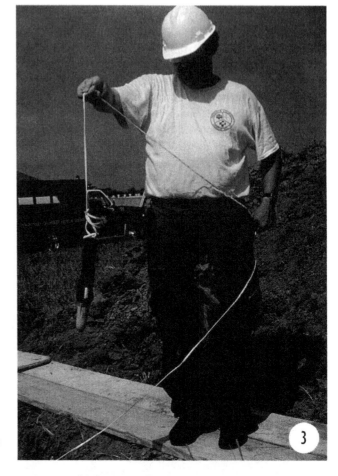

Step 2. Lay down 4- by 8-foot panels next to the trench lip on the side of the trench opposite the spoil pile. These panels should be placed end to end so that there is a continuous walkway and should extend for several feet on each side of the affected area. ▲

Step 3. Monitor the atmospheric conditions in the trench. ▶

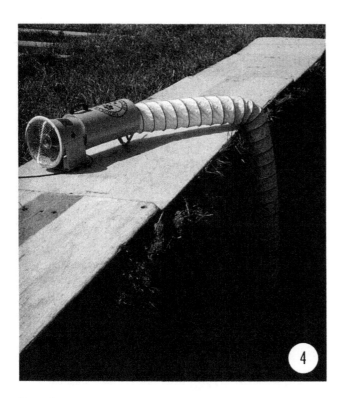

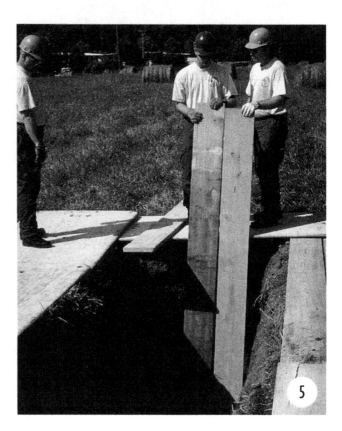

Step 4. Ventilate the trench. ▲

Step 5. "Safe" the end of the trench. ▲

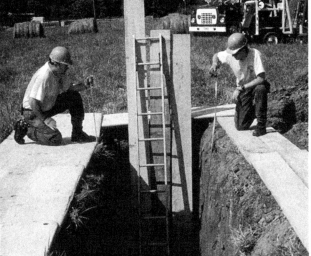

Step 6. Measure the depth of the trench on both sides. ◀

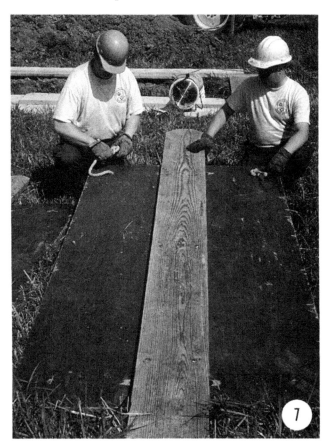

Step 7. Secure the ropes to the panels, if necessary. ▶

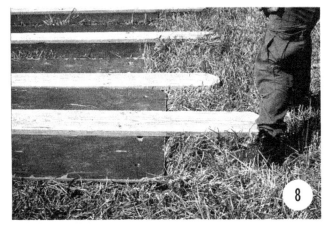

◀ ▼
Step 8. Place the prefabricated panels side by side, and even, if the floor of the trench is level. Adjust the position of the panels if the trench floor is not level. Nail the scabs that will support the shores. Secure each scab with two nails. Position the scabs so that the shores will be evenly spaced throughout the depth of the trench, but in no case position the scabs so that the shores will be more than 4 feet apart.

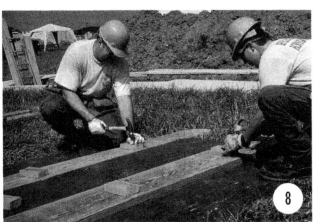

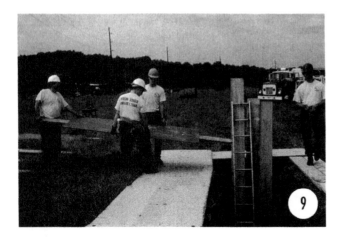

Step 9. Turn one panel over and lower it into the trench with the upright facing in. ◄

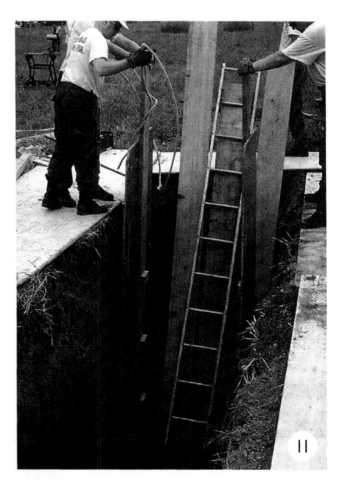

Step 10. Pass the ropes to rescuers on the opposite side of the trench. Adjust the panel so that it stands vertically against the trench wall.

Step 11. While one rescuer holds the first panel in place, lower the second panel into the trench with the upright facing in. Make sure that the panels are directly opposite each other, and that each panel is snug against the trench wall and vertical. The two rescuers should continue to hold the panels vertically against the trench walls during the shoring operation, preventing the panels from slipping sideways. ▲

Step 12. Make sure that the ladder is close to the working area so that the rescuer installing the first shore will not have to reach over an unsafe distance.

Step 13. Climb down the ladder, but no deeper into the trench than waist-level. This will minimize the possibility of being completely buried in the event of a secondary cave-in. Measure the distance between the uprights at the top set of scabs.

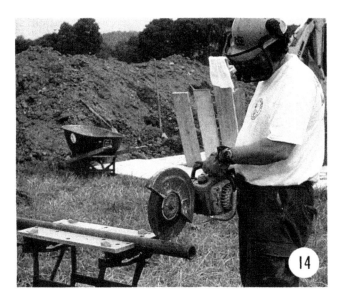

Step 14. Cut a length of pipe to the measurement between the uprights less 8 inches. The 8 inches allows for room taken up by the screw-jack ends. ◄

▶

Step 15. Place the ends of the assembled shore on the top set of scabs. It is important that you shore the first set of panels from the top down when using screw jacks, just as it is when using timbers. When the top shore is in place, there will be little chance for a secondary wall collapse or additional spoil-pile movement.

Step 16. Turn the handles of the jack to lengthen the shore and thus tighten it against the uprights. Do not overtighten; to do so may cause the bottom of each panel to move inward.

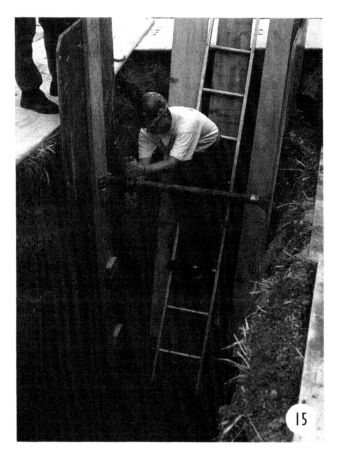

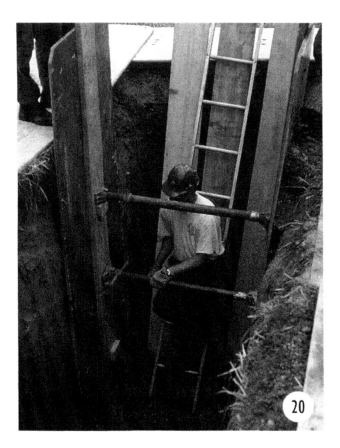

Step 17. Secure the ends of the shore to the uprights with nails through the holes provided.

Step 18. Climb down the ladder and measure the distance between the uprights at the middle set of scabs.

Step 19. Cut a length of pipe for the second shore. Remember to cut the pipe 8 inches less than the measurement between the uprights.

Step 20. Secure the middle shore with nails. Tighten it with the nut handles. ◄

Step 21. Prepare the bottom shore in the same way.

Step 22. Place and secure the bottom shore by nailing it in place and tightening it with the nut handles. ▶

Step 23. When all of the shores are nailed in place and tentatively tightened, make them snug with a "cheater," a short length of pipe that provides additional leverage.

> ### Remember
> You can exert considerable force with a cheater pipe. Be careful that you do not split the uprights.

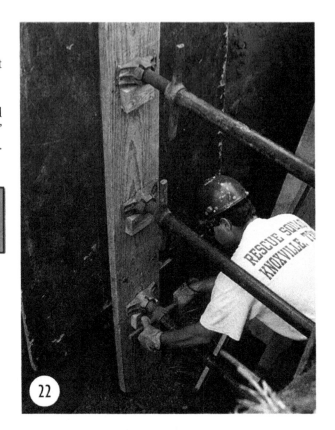

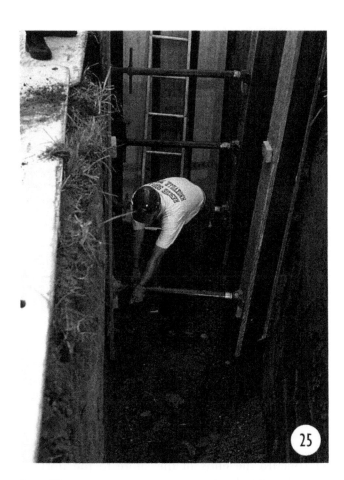

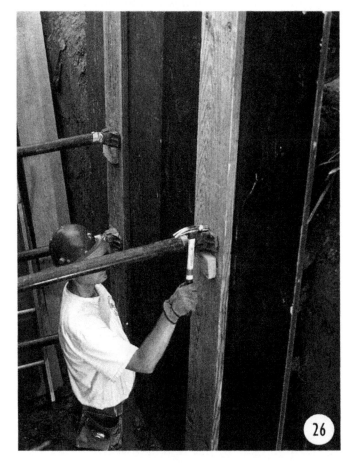

Step 24. Position the second set of panels directly next to the first set. As when shoring with timbers, the rescuer in the trench can assist with the placement since he is working from a safe area.

Step 25. Position the bottom shore against the second set of panels. Keep in mind that it is not necessary to shore from the top down once the first set of panels is in place. Since this trench is 8 feet deep, it will require only two shores. (For safety's sake, always start with at least three.) ▲

Step 26. As the shoring of the second set of panels nears completion, a rescuer can begin to fill in voids between the panels and the walls of the trench with dirt from the spoil pile.

Step 27. Using the same sequence, install the third set of panels, bottom shore first. ▶

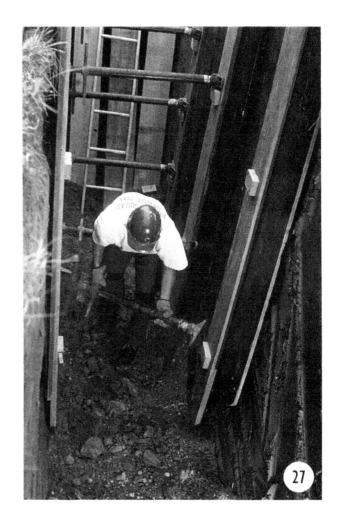

◀

Step 28. Finally, install the top shore.

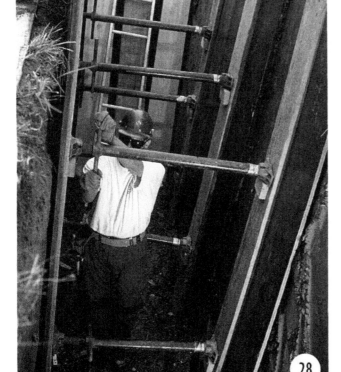

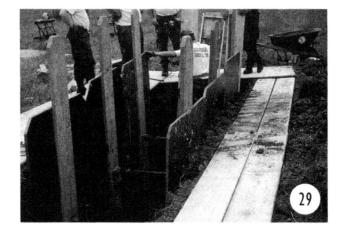

Step 29. Remove any debris that may interfere with the digging operation. Be sure that the blower continues to operate. ▲

USING SHEETING AND PNEUMATIC SHORING

Speed and efficiency can be increased by using pneumatic shoring. There is no need to nail scabs on the uprights; nor is there any need for boxing and wedging the shoring in place as there is with timber shoring and screw jacks. An important advantage of pneumatic shores is that they can be safely installed when trench walls are angled.

Measure the width and depth of the trench so that you can determine the size and amount of the shores you will need.

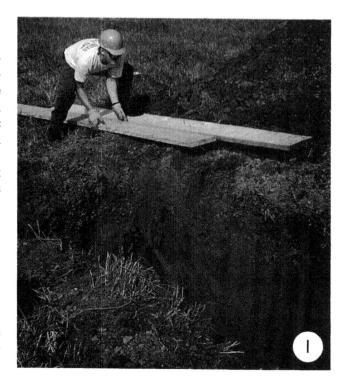

Step 1. Level the ground between the edge of the trench and the body of the spoil pile and lay down 2- by 12-inch planks. These planks will serve as ground pads. ▶

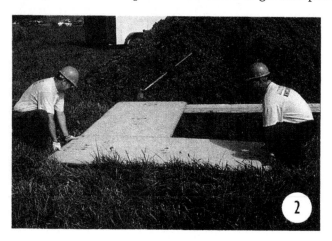

◀
Step 2. Lay down 4- by 8-foot panels next to the trench lip on the side of the trench opposite the spoil pile. These panels should be placed end to end so that there is a continuous walkway and should extend for several feet on each side of the affected area.

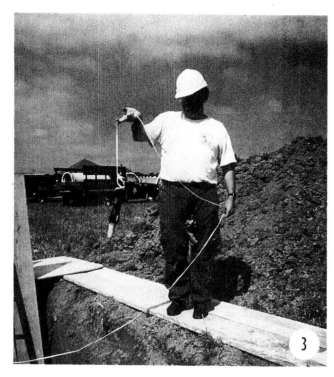

Step 3. Monitor the atmospheric conditions in the trench. ▶

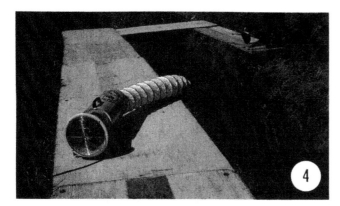

Step 4. Ventilate the trench.

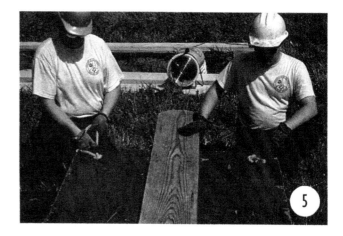

Step 5. Secure ropes to the panels, if necessary. ▶

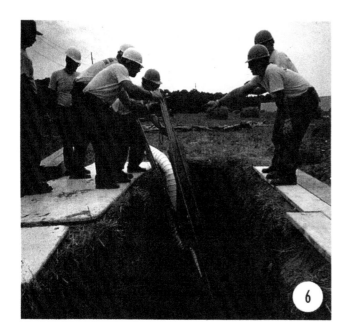

Step 6. Turn one panel over and lower it into the trench with the upright facing in. ◀

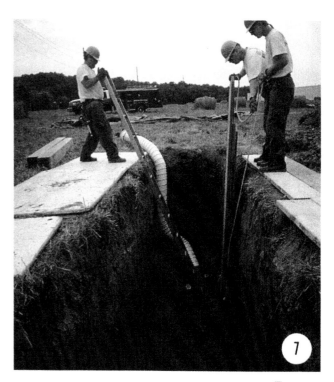

Step 7. Pass the ropes to rescuers on the opposite side of the trench. Adjust the panel so that it stands vertically against the trench wall. ▶

Step 8. While one rescuer holds the first panel in place, lower the second panel into the trench with the upright facing in. Make sure that the panels are directly opposite each other, and that each panel is snug against the trench wall and vertical. Two rescuers should continue to hold the panels vertically against the trench walls during the shoring operation so that they can prevent the panels from slipping sideways. ▶

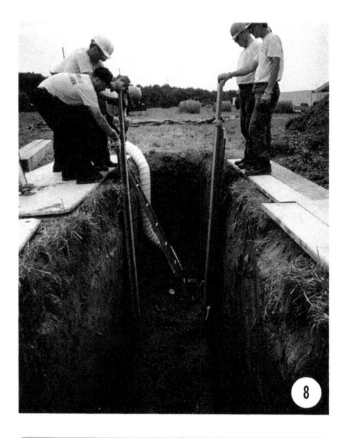

Note
It will be necessary to lower the first shore into the trench with a rope. Instead of tying the rope around the shore in the manner suggested for timbers and screw jacks, make up a lowering - line and hook combination like the one shown in Figure 4-17. The hook is made from a welding rod, and the eye is formed in the rope by passing the end through the strands in two places.

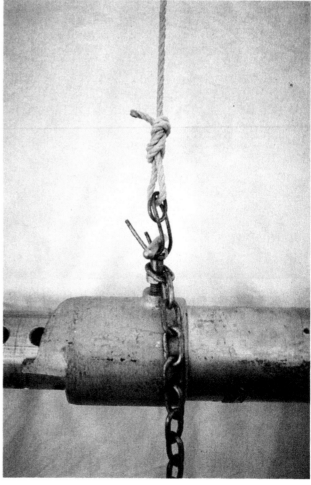

Figure 4-17. A lowering line and hook.

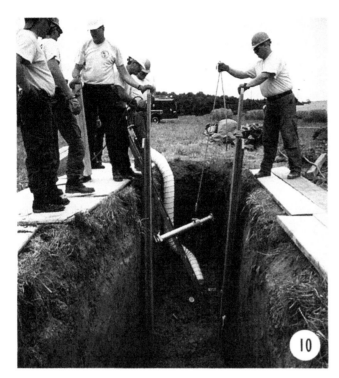

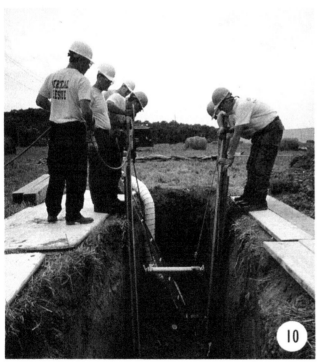

Step 9. Attach the quick coupler of the air supply hose to the nipple of an appropriate-sized jack. Place the double hook of the lowering line under the T-handle. Tighten the T-handle slightly so that the collar will not pull free from the body of the shore while it is being lowered.

Step 10. Lower the shore into the trench using two rescuers. One rescuer lowers one side of the jack with the air hose, while the second rescuer lowers the other side with the rope and hook. If the trench is less than 4 feet wide, the lowering operation can be accomplished by one rescuer. The base of the shore is positioned against the center of the upright so that the piston end can move against the opposite upright.◀

If the trench is over 4 feet wide, tie a line on the nipple end of the jack for lowering purposes, because the shore will be too heavy to support with the air hose.

In this 8-foot deep trench the first shore is lowered 4 feet, or halfway into the trench. Shoring is begun at the midpoint, rather than at the top of the panels, as suggested for shoring with timber and screw jacks. The load-bearing capability of pneumatic shoring makes this practical. Also, because of the spreading forces generated with pneumatic shoring, placing the first shore at the top of a pair of panels may cause the bottom of the panels to kick in. ◀

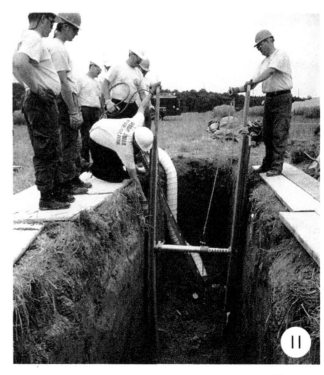

Step 11. Instruct the rescuer operating the air valve to pressurize the jack. ▶

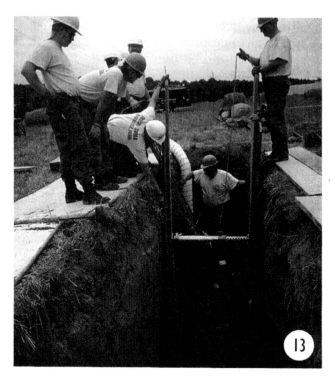

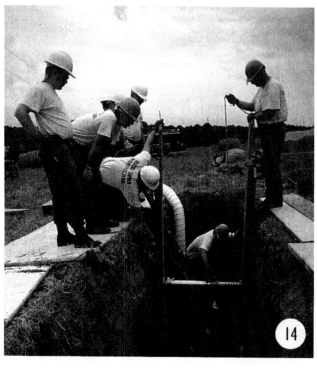

Step 12. Place a ladder in the trench. Adjust the ladder to accommodate the person entering the trench.

Step 13. Climb down the ladder and disconnect the rope hook from the T-handle. Lock the shore in its extended position by inserting the pin, rotating the collar until it is snugly seated against the pin, and tightening the T-handle. When this is accomplished, instruct the rescuer operating the air valve to release the pressure, and remove the coupler from the jack. ◄

Step 14. For safety, drive nails through the end plates of the shore into the uprights. This will prevent the shore from falling if it becomes loose as other shores are installed. ▲

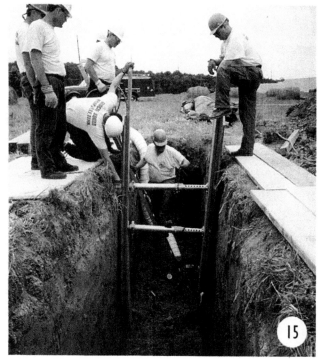

Step 15. Couple the air hose to another shore, and hand the shore to the rescuer on the ladder. ◄

Step 16. Install this shore at a point 2 feet below the trench lip.

Step 17. Lock the shore in place and secure it with nails.

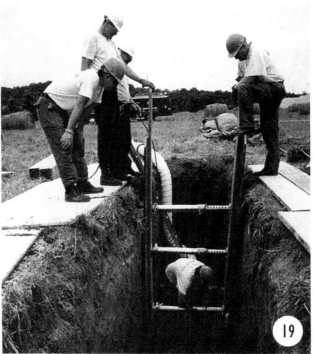

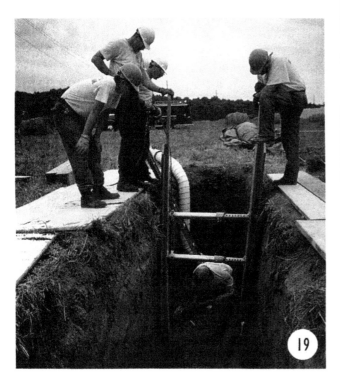

Step 18 Couple another shore to the air hose and pass it to the rescuer on the ladder.

Step 19. Install the shore at the 6-foot level. ◀ ▲

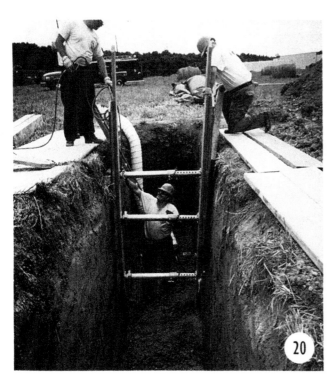

Step 20. Check the shores to make sure that none have become loose while the others were being installed. Readjust if necessary. ◀

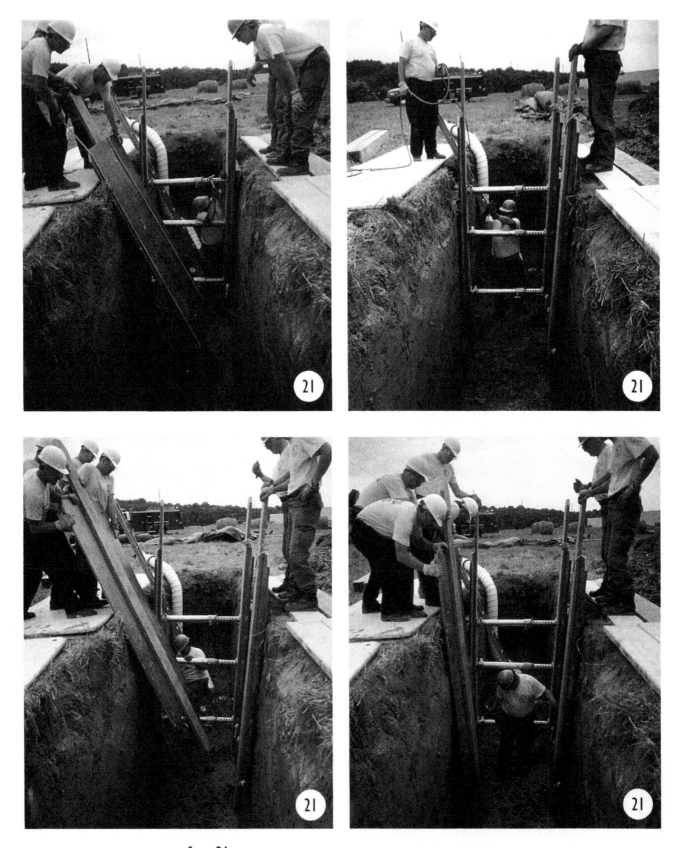

Step 21. Place another pair of panels in the trench.

Step 22. Because this trench is only 8 feet deep, after the first set of panels use only two shores. Place one shore at the 2-foot level and the second shore at the 6-foot level.

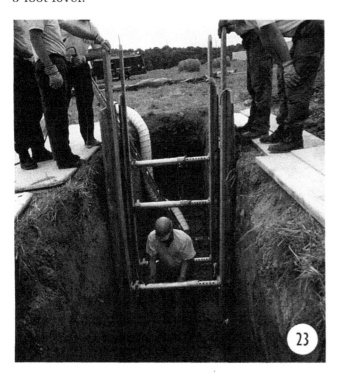

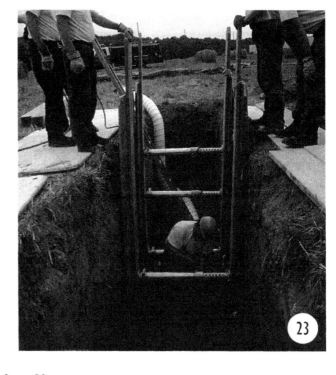

Step 23. Install the bottom shore at the 6-foot level since the rescuer is already in position. ◄ ▲

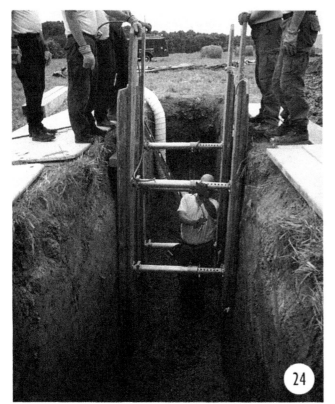

Step 24. Depending on the height of the installer, you may need a second ladder in the trench next to the second pair of panels. Install the top shore at the 2-foot level. Do not forget the safety nails. ◄ ▼

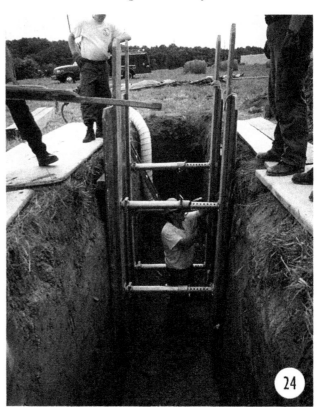

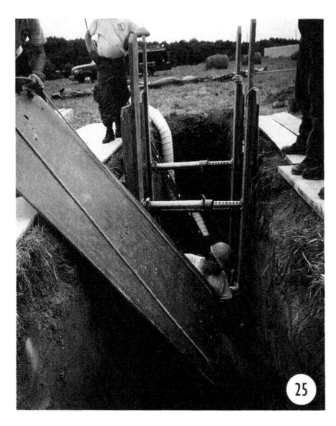

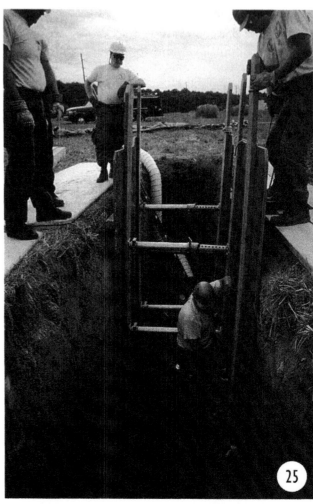

Step 25. Position additional pairs of panels in the same way. ▲ ▶

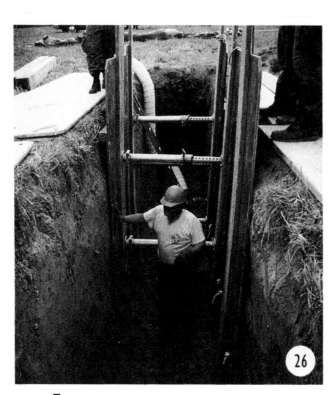

Step 26. Remember to have a rescuer hold the first panel vertically and firmly against the trench wall while the second panel is being placed. ◀

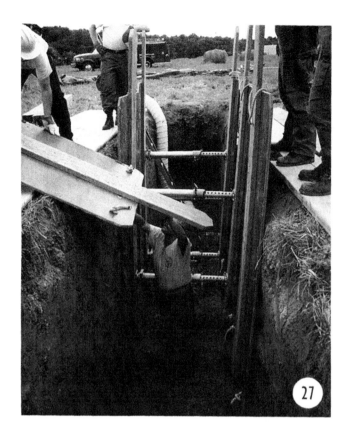

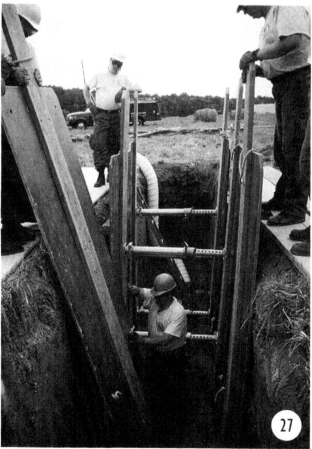

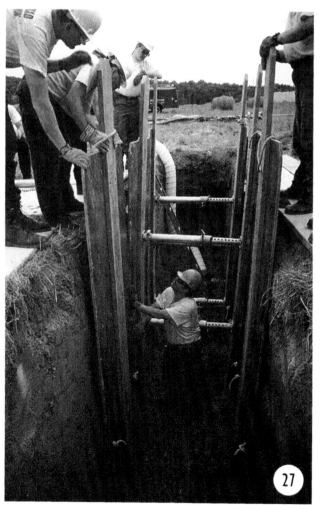

Step 27. The rescuer in the trench can assist with the placing of additional panels since he is now working from a safe area. ◀▼

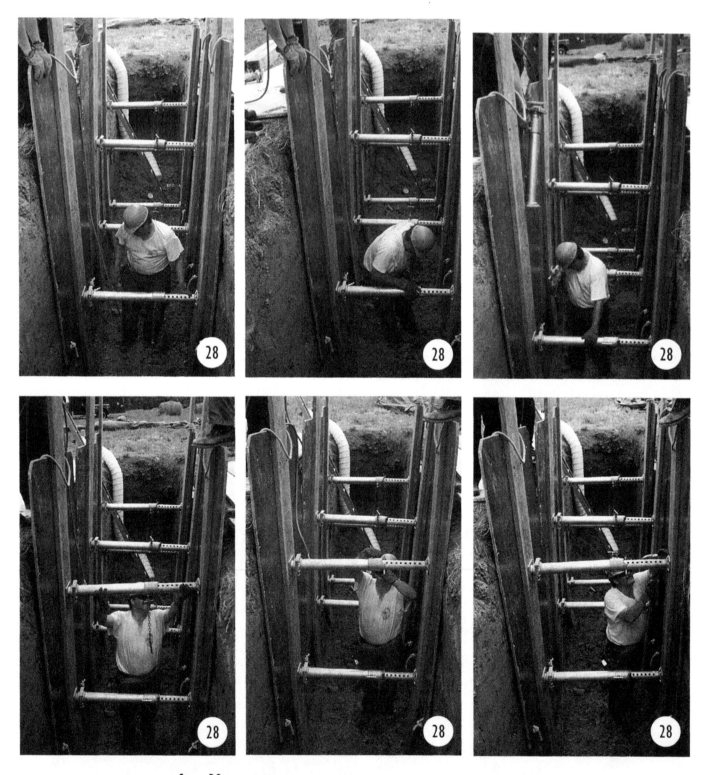

Step 28. Install the shores in the same order as the second pair: first the bottom and finally the top.

Step 29. Fill in any voids that exist between the sheeting and the trench walls.

Step 30. Remove debris and tools from the trench and keep the blower operating.

TRENCH WALL COLLAPSE— ONE SIDE

In the three situations just discussed, the trench walls remained nearly vertical and provided a base for the sheeting. In the case of a trench wall collapse, you will find that an entire section of the trench wall has caved in (Figure 4-18). A void has been created and there is no longer an earth foundation against which the sheeting can be supported.

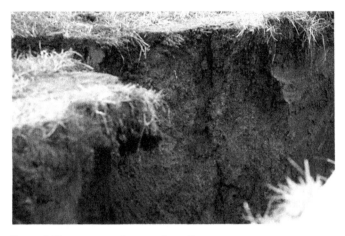

Figure 4-18. A one-side trench collapse.

Therefore, it will be necessary to create an "artificial" foundation. This can be done with a heavy timber, which is referred to as a wale. Instead of a timber, however, you can use a 24-foot extension ladder as a wale. This ladder is generally carried on an engine or truck, and, besides being readily available, it is strong enough to serve as a foundation. Do not use a painter's ladder as a wale in wall-collapse situations because painter's ladders lack the strength of fire department ladders. This situation calls for the use of timbers, screw jacks, or pneumatic shores.

Using sheeting and pneumatic shoring. The area close to the trench is prepared in much the same way as in the situations discussed earlier. Extra care must be taken while placing ground panels around the collapsed portion, however, to prevent additional cave-in. Though a step-by-step method for sheeting and shoring operations is presented, many of the steps should be done simultaneously. Instructions are given for sheeting and shoring with pneumatic shores. The instructions and steps are the same for using timbers and screw jacks; however, these take longer to place and require the use of scabs.

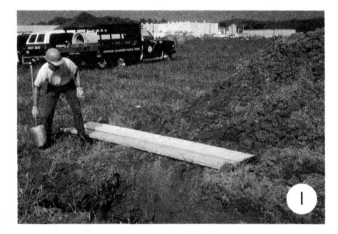

Step 1. Level the ground between the edge of the trench and the body of the spoil pile to accept the 2- by 12-inch planks that will serve as ground pads. Stand on a two-by-twelve as you level the ground, then slide the plank forward. Do this every 3 feet. ▶

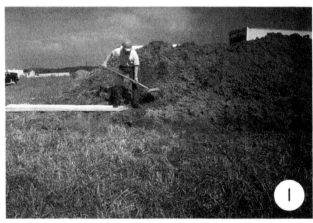

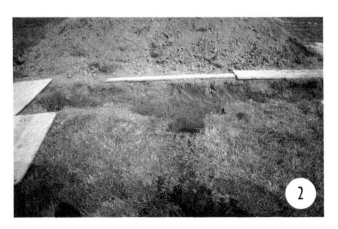

Step 2. Place the 2- by 12-inch planks with their ends as close to the edge of the caved-in area as possible.

Step 3. Lay down 4- by 8-foot panels next to the trench lip on the side of the trench opposite the spoil pile. These panels should be placed end to end so that there is a continuous walkway along the trench lip. The panels should extend for a few feet on each side of the affected area. When the collapse involves the side of the trench opposite the spoil pile, the ends of the 4- by 8-foot panels should be placed as close to the void edge as possible. ▶

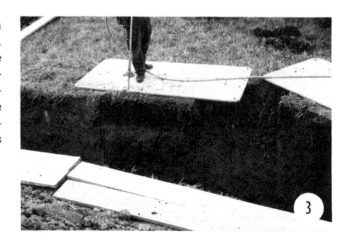

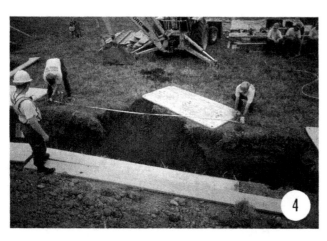

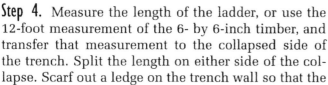

Step 4. Measure the length of the ladder, or use the 12-foot measurement of the 6- by 6-inch timber, and transfer that measurement to the collapsed side of the trench. Split the length on either side of the collapse. Scarf out a ledge on the trench wall so that the ladder or timber will fit into it and on the ledge, even with the side of the trench. The idea is to keep the ladder or timber from protruding into the trench and allowing a void between the trench wall and the sheeting. This ledge can be made easily with an air knife, or a bar or spade. ▲ ▼

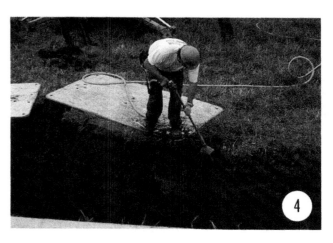

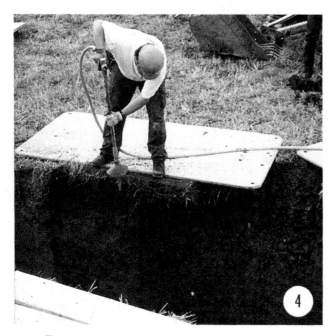

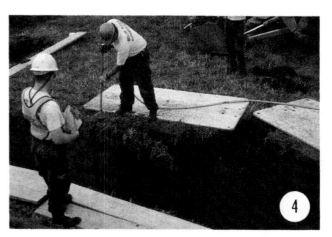

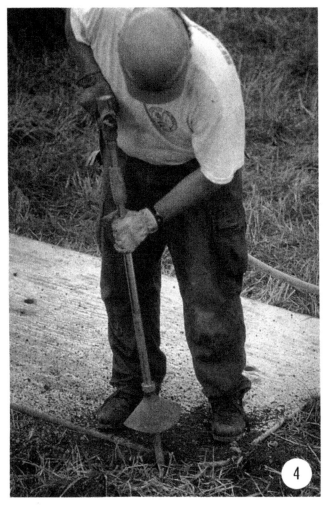

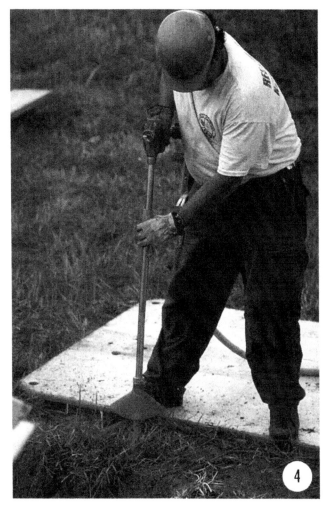

Step 4. Continued ▲ ▶ ▼

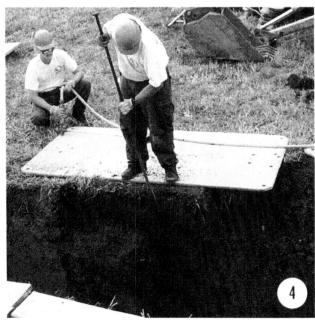

Step 5. Span the caved-in area with the 6-inch by 6-inch by 12-foot timber. ▶

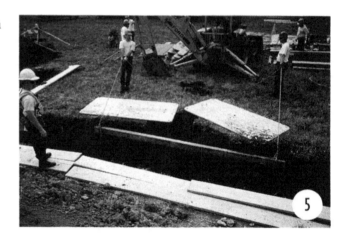

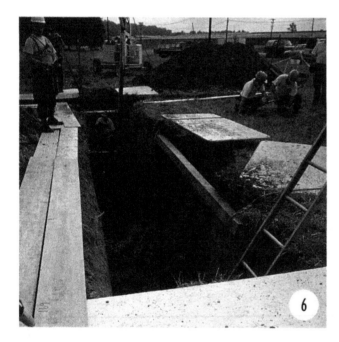

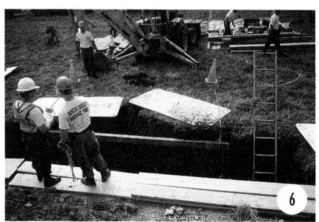

Step 6. Lower the timber 2 to 3 feet into the trench. The rescuers lowering the timber with the ropes will be responsible for maintaining the timber in position until it is held in place with sheeting and shoring. Note that the timber sits on the ledge formed in Step 4. Two stakes can be driven 10 feet back from the trench. The ropes to the timber can be tied off on them, relieving the two rescuers who are holding the ropes. ◀ ▲

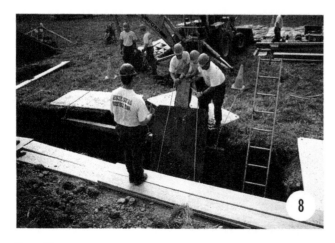

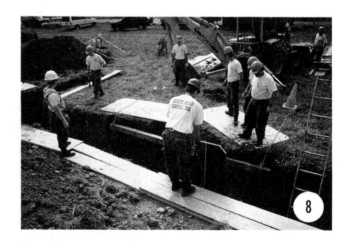

Step 7. Secure ropes to the panels.

Step 8. Place the first panel in the trench so that the upright faces in. Have a rescuer continue to hold the panel. ▲ ◀

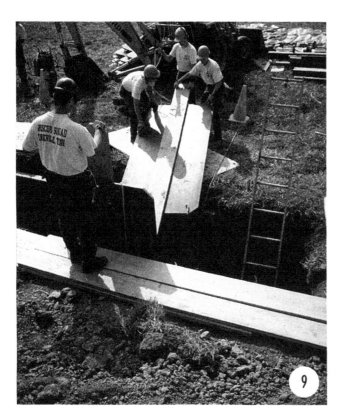

Step 9. Place a second panel opposite the first. ◀

Step 10. Place a ladder in the trench, monitor the atmospheric conditions, and set up the blower for ventilation.

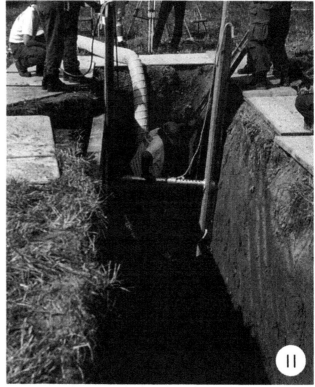

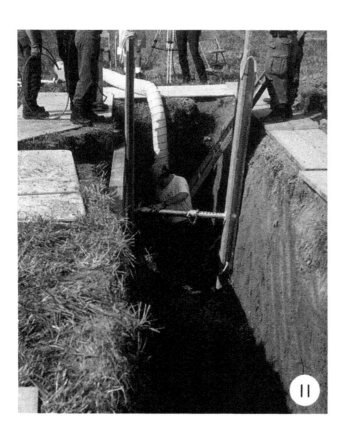

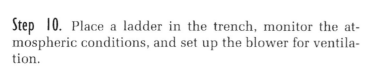

◀▲
Step 11. Hook up and pressurize the first shore midway in the trench. Secure it with safety nails.

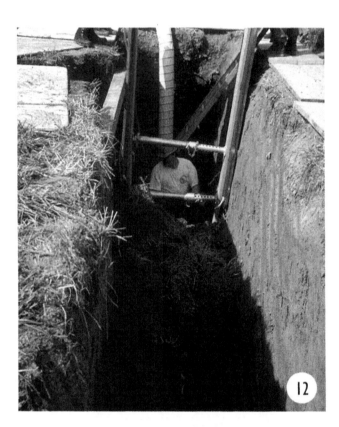

Step 12. Place the bottom shore. ◄

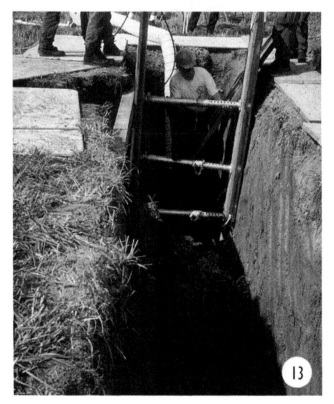

Step 13. Place the top shore. ◄ ▼

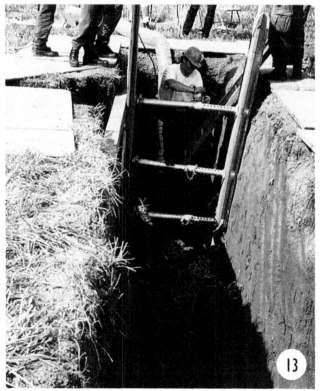

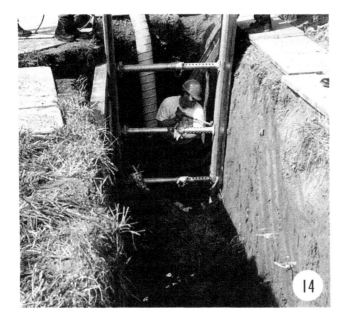

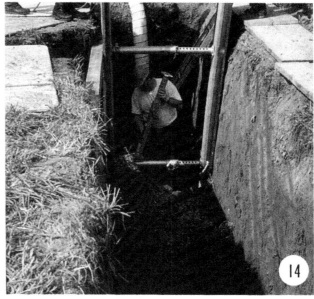

Step 14. Since we need only two shores in the 8-foot-deep trench, remove the center shore. We now have a safe area to work in because the sheeting pins the outside wale to the trench wall. ▲▼▲▼

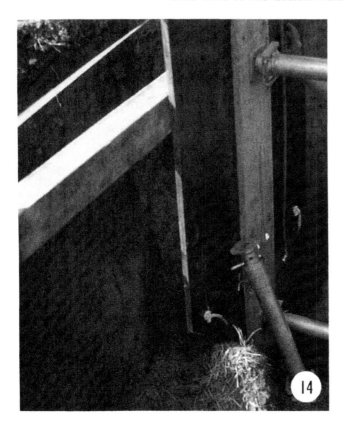

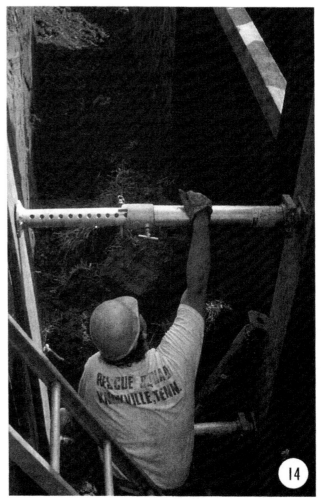

Step 15. Proceed to make another safe area on the other side of the cave-in. Measure over $4\frac{1}{2}$ feet to place the second pair of panels. Make sure to leave a few inches between panels, rather than overlapping them. You can have up to a foot between panels, but it is better to maintain the close sheeting. ▶

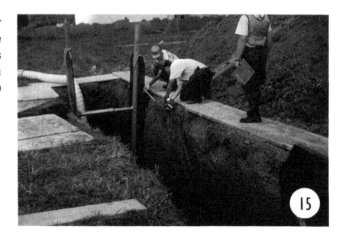

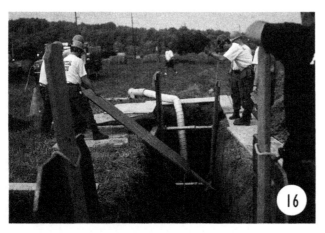

Step 16. Place another panel in the trench on the side opposite the cave-in. Have a rescuer hold it. ▲ ▶

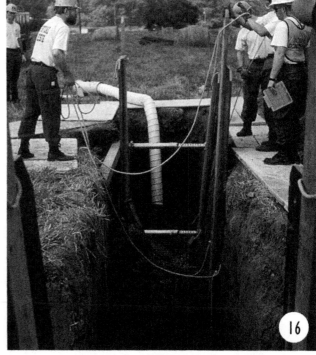

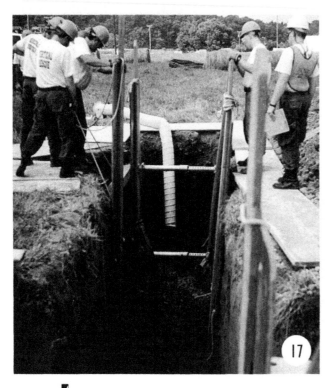

Step 17. Place the second panel and line it up with the first.

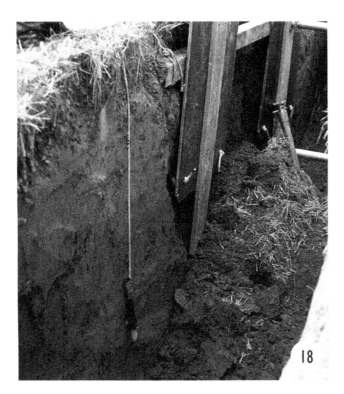

Step 18. Keep ventilating the trench, and continue to take readings from the monitor. ◄

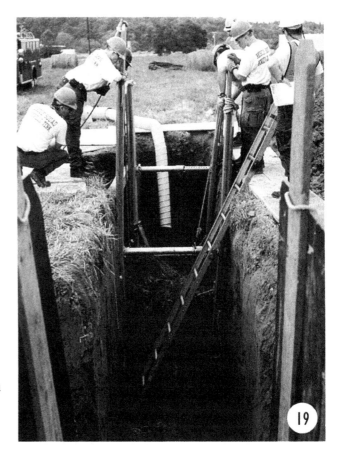

Step 19. Hang the center shore and pressurize it. Place a ladder in the trench. ▶

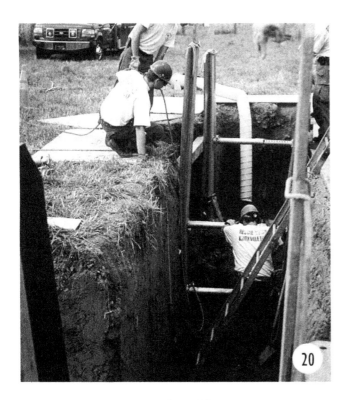

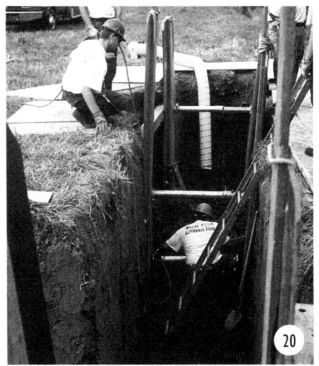

Step 20. Secure the center shore, then place the bottom and top shores. ▲ ▲

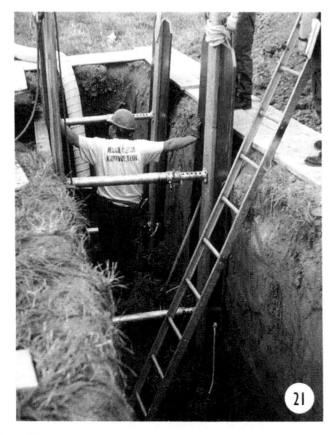

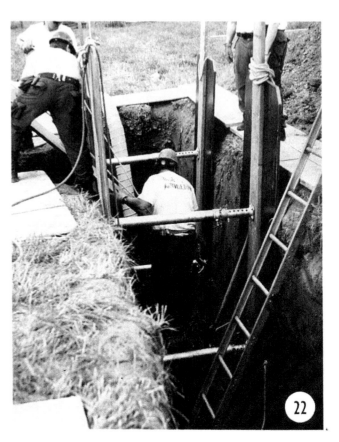

Step 21. Remove the center shore because it is not needed in the 8-foot trench. ▲

Step 22. Place another set of panels in the collapsed area. Position the far side first. ▲

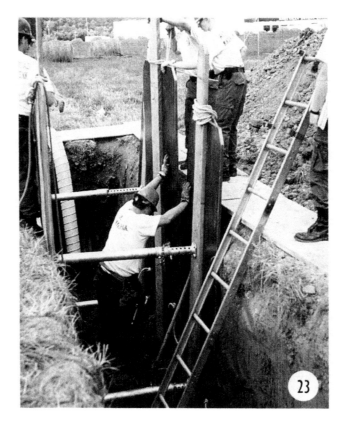

Step 23. Have a rescuer on top hold the panels in place. ▲

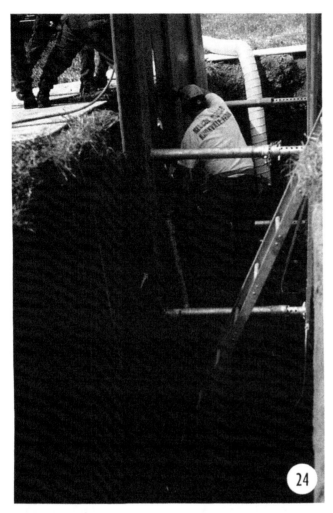

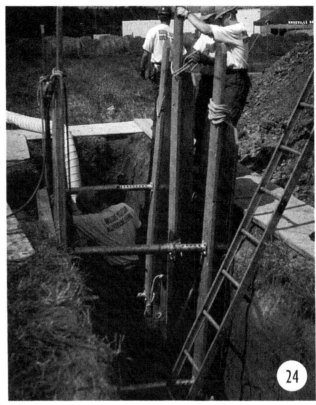

Step 24. Position the caved-in side next. Note how the timber placed against the outside wale acts as the trench wall. ◀ ◀ ▲

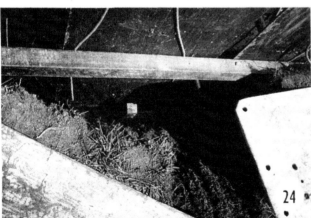

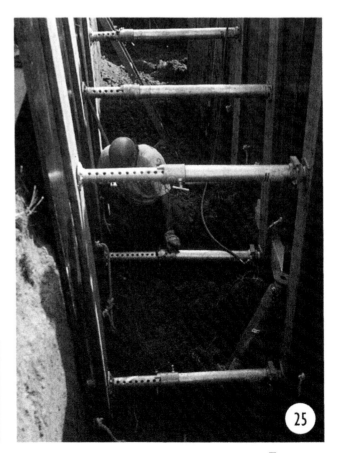

Step 25. You can now place the bottom and top shores. It does not matter in which order as long as there is a solid base behind the panels. ▶

Note
Whenever you install a pneumatic shore against a base that is over a void, "feather" (or gently operate) the valve so that the jack lengthens slowly. This prevents the full force of the shore from being exerted all at once and will prevent possible damage to the sheeting panel.

Step 26. The final result is a solid-walled trench prepared for rescue work or extensive digging. ▶

Step 27. If you must go deeper, it is time to install the walers and supplemental shoning. We will cover these steps later. ▶

> **Note**
> Whenever you install a pneumatic shore against a base that is over a void, "frather" (or gently operate) the valve, so that the jack lengthens slowly. This prevents the full force of the shore from being exerted all at once and will prevent possible damage to the sheeting panel.

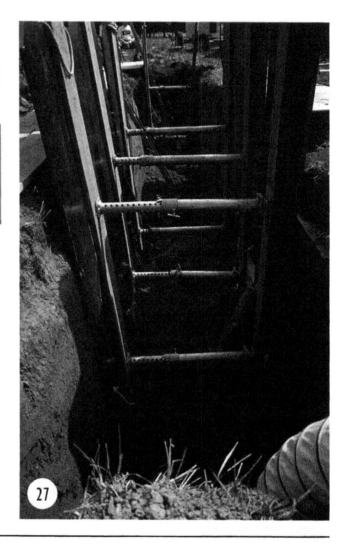

TRENCH WALL COLLAPSE— BOTH SIDES

In this situation you will find that a section of both trench walls has caved in. (Figure 4-19). Two voids have been created, and there are no longer firm foundations against which the sheeting can be supported. It will be necessary, then, to create two artificial foundations. Again, 24-foot extension ladders or 6- by 6-inch timbers can serve effectively as wales. We will be using the 6-inch by 6-inch by 12-foot timbers as both inside and outside wales. Preparation of the ground is extremely important in this operation. The rescuers must have a safe environment in which to effectively complete the rescue operation.

Using sheeting and pneumatic shores. Again, the procedure is essentially the same as for shoring with timbers and screw jacks.

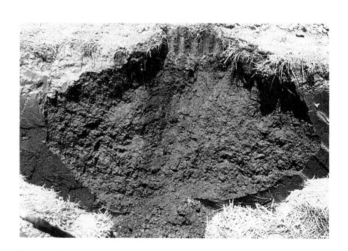

Figure 4-19. A double-side cave-in.

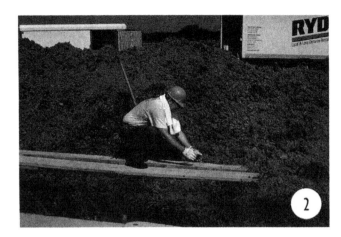

Step 1. Level the ground between the edge of the trench and the spoil pile.

Step 2. Place 2- by 12-inch ground planks close to the trench lip, with their ends as close to the collapsed area as possible. ◄

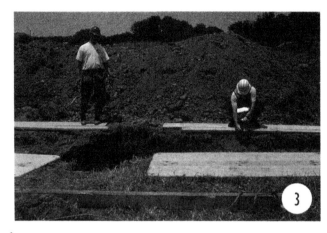

Step 3. Lay down 4- by 8-foot ground pads parallel to the trench, with their edges close to the edges of the collapsed area. Measure and mark for the placement of the outside wales. ►

Step 4. Monitor the atmosphere in the trench, and set up the fresh air blower for ventilation.

Step 5. Tie ropes to the panels.

◄

Step 6. Cut away dirt on trench sidewalls to form a ledge for the outside wales. Use the air knife and/or bar.

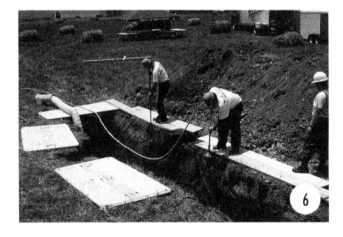

Step 7. Position the wales on the ledges of both sides of the trench with ropes. ►

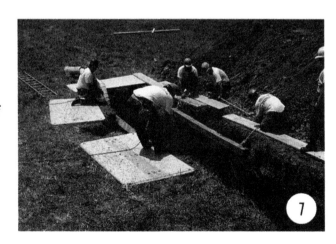

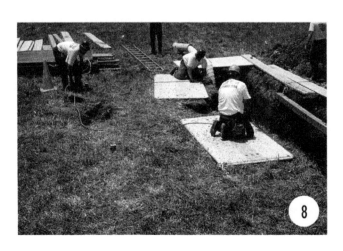

Step 8. Drive stakes into the ground to hold the ropes so that rescuers are free to do other tasks. ◄

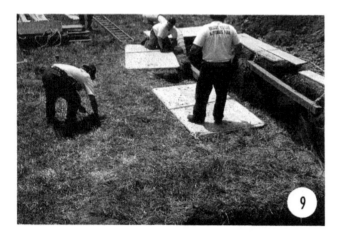

Step 10. Place the first panel near one end of the cave-in. ▶

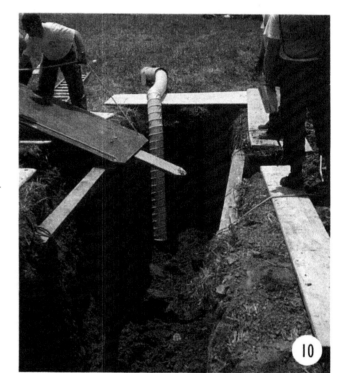

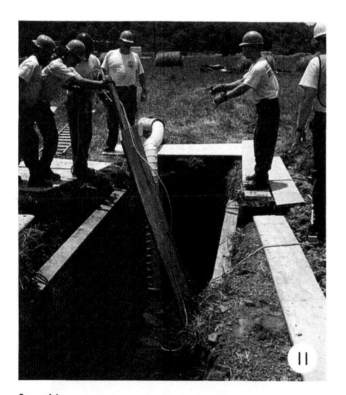

Step 11. Push the panel over to the opposite side. ▲

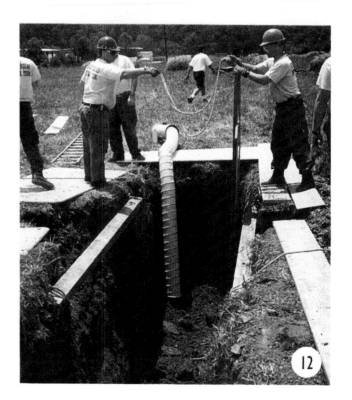

Step 12. Have a rescuer hold the panel in place. ▶

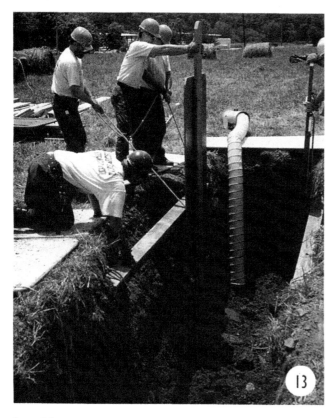

Step 13. Place the second panel. ▲

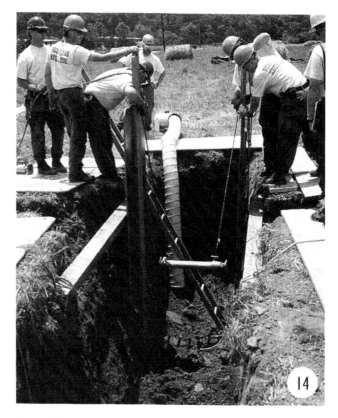

Step 14. Suspend the appropriate-sized shore between the uprights. ▲

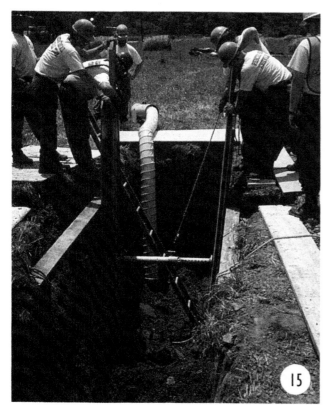

Step 15. Pressurize the shore. ▲

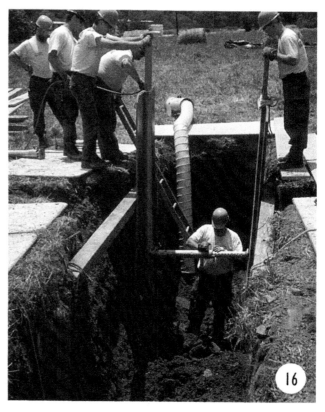

Step 16. Descend the ladder and secure the shore. ▲

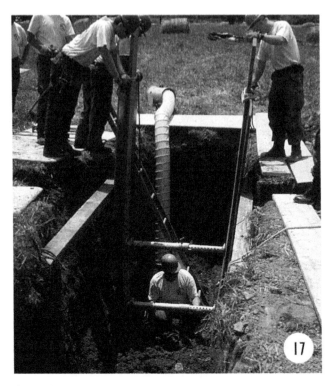

Step 17. Install the bottom shore. ▲

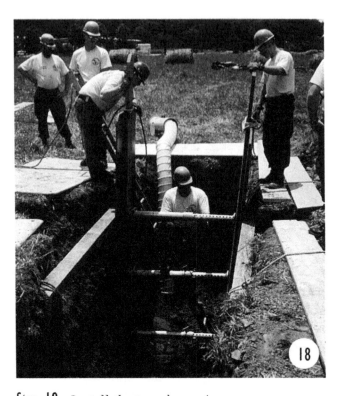

Step 18. Install the top shore. ▲

Step 19. Remove the center shore since it is not needed in the 8-foot-deep trench.

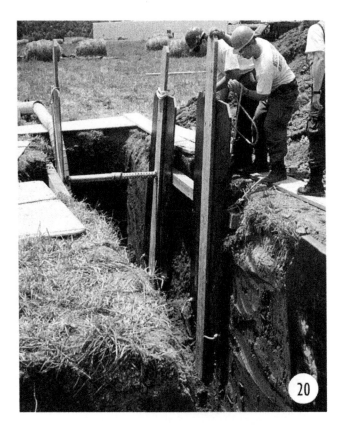

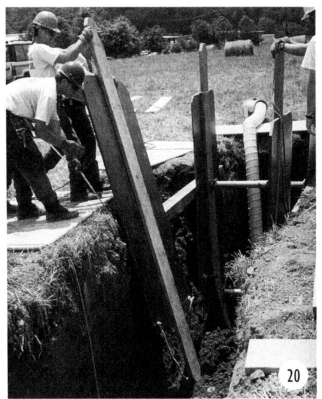

Step 20. Place another pair of panels at the other end of the collapsed area. ▲ ▲

Step 21. Place a ladder in the trench. ▶

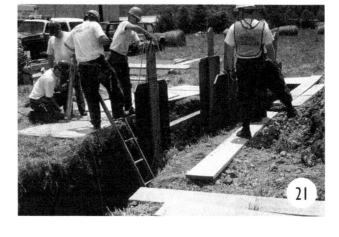

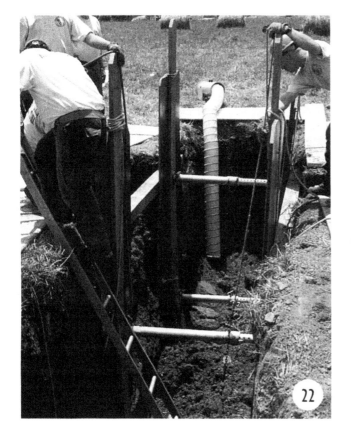

Step 22. Install a shore between the uprights at about the center of the trench. ◀ ▼

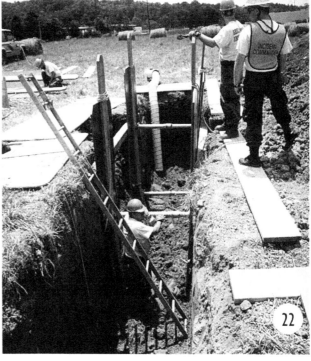

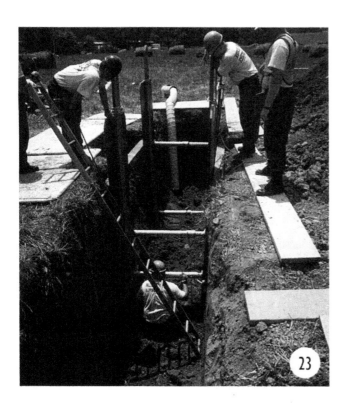

Step 23. Install the bottom shore. ◀

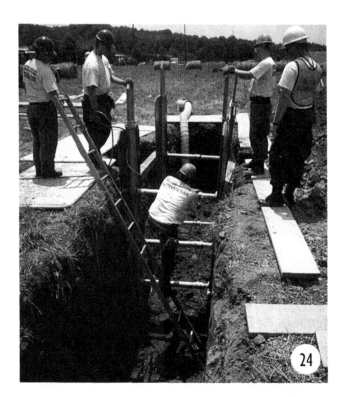

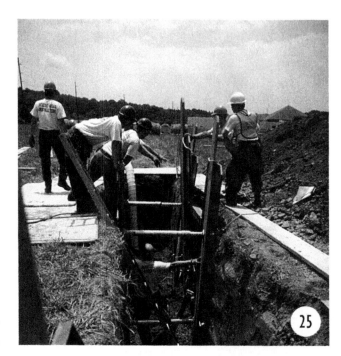

Step 24. Install the third shore. There are now two safe areas from which rescuers can work. ◄

Step 25. Remove the center shore. ►

Step 26. Place the fifth panel in the center. ◄

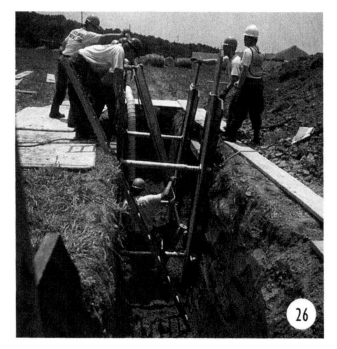

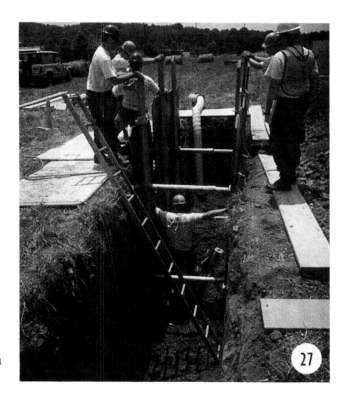

Step 27. Finally, place the sixth panel opposite the fifth to fill in the caved-in area. ►

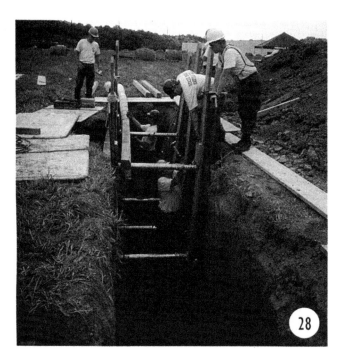

Step 28. Nail 2- by 12- by 12-inch scabs on the uprights before placing the inside wales. The wales will butt up against the scabs and assure the correct spacing for supplemental sheeting (as covered in Phase 8 under "Supplemental Sheeting and Shoring"). ◀

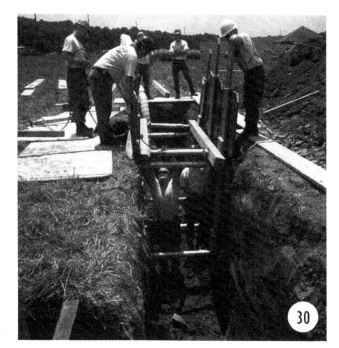

Step 29. Place the inside wales across the shores. Position hem evenly and make certain that they are not locking in the shoring by trapping the end lip.

Step 30. Pressurize one end of the shore and then the other. ▶

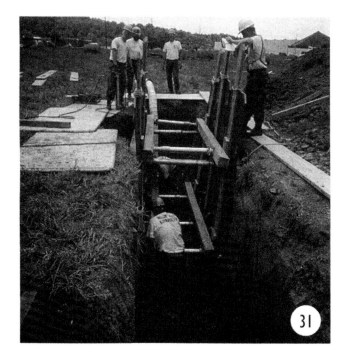

Step 31. Place bottom walers. ◀

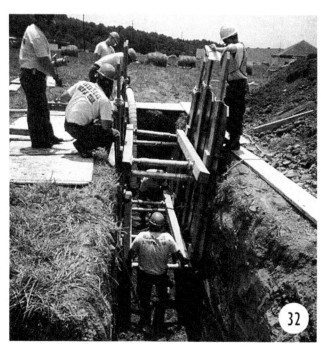

Step 32. Pressurize one end of the shore making sure that the wales are level opposite each other. It does not matter if they are not level end to end. ▶

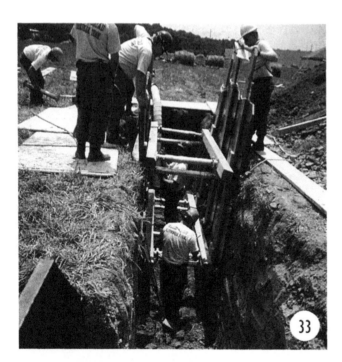

Step 33. Once one end is secure, you can level the wales using them as levers. Now pressurize the other end. ◄

Step 34. Remove both center shores. This allows ample room for digging. ►

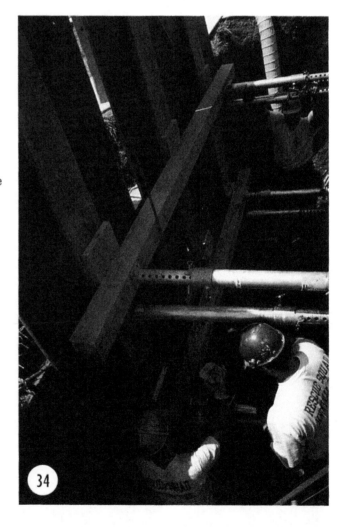

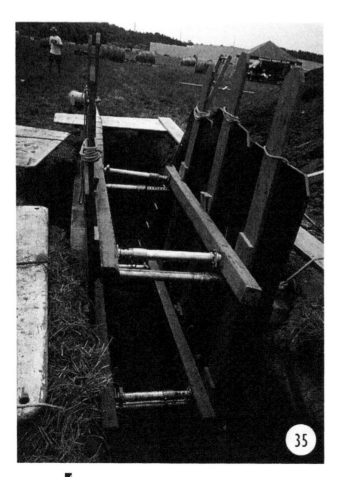

Step 35. The task is now complete. We are ready to dig or install supplemental sheeting and shoring. ◄

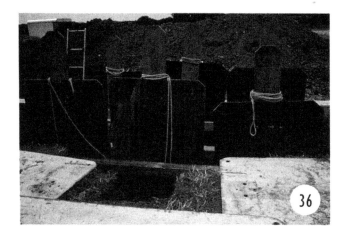

Step 36. Note how the outside wale provides a solid wall for the sheeting. ◄

Step 37. All openings are filled with wedges to prevent any movement of the sheeting. ▶

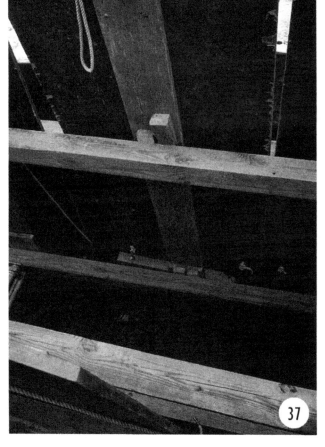

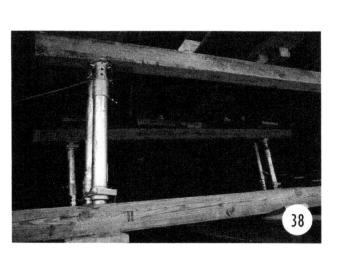

Step 38. Remove debris from the floor of the trench in preparation for the digging effort. Be sure to keep the blower operating during the sheeting and shoring procedures, and continue to monitor the atmosphere. Keep in mind that all the shores not holding the wales can be removed if they are needed elsewhere. However, if they are not needed, you should leave them in place so that you will not have to put them back in to remove the structure. ◄

SHORING THE "T" TRENCH

As we proceed with the next few operations, we will again only illustrate the pneumatic shores. Instructions for the placement and use of timber shoring and screw jacks are the same. Preparation for the operation remains the same, so we will list the preliminary steps in abbreviated form.

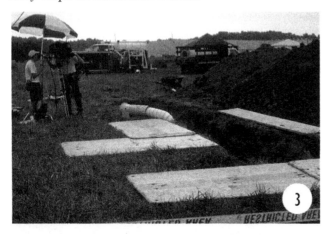

Step 1. Level all surfaces for ground planks.

Step 2. Place the ground planks.

Step 3. Lay down the ground pads as shown. ◄

Step 4. Monitor the trench for atmospheric conditions.

Step 5. Set up the blower and ventilate the trench.

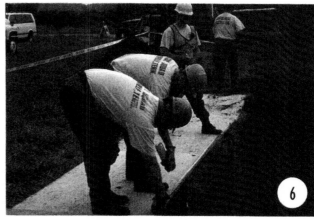

Step 6. It is critical to measure all operations from here on so that the corners will be tight, without overlaps. ►

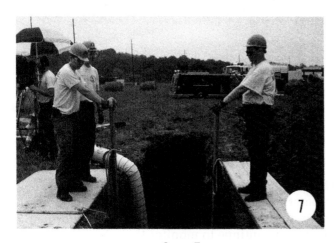

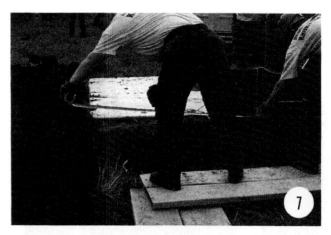

Step 7. Position the first set of panels 4 feet back from the intercepting leg of the "T." The object is to establish a "safe zone" to work from that is far enough away from the dangerous corners should they collapse. Make sure that the exact distance is checked so that the next set of panels will not extend into the "T." ▲ ▲

Step 8. Hang the shore. ◄

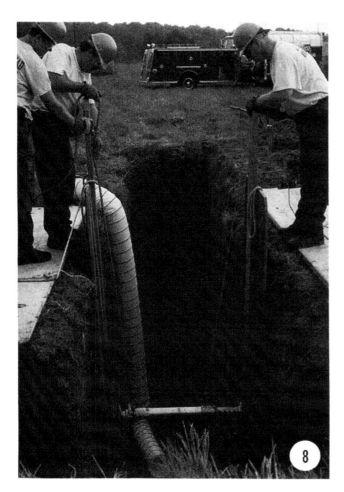

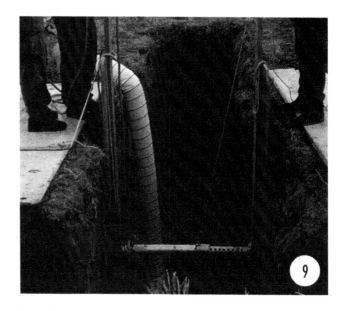

Step 9. Pressurize the shore. ▲

Step 10. Secure the safety nails. ◄

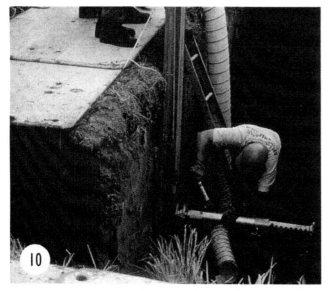

Step 11. Place the top shore and then the bottom shore. This procedure can be reversed if there is no backing on the top shore. In that case, pressurize the bottom shore first, back up the top of the panel with an appropriately sized timber (4- by 4-inch or 6- by 6-inch), and then place the top shore. Keep in mind that when you are sheeting and shoring a trench, you must remain flexible in your thinking while not compromising safety. ▶

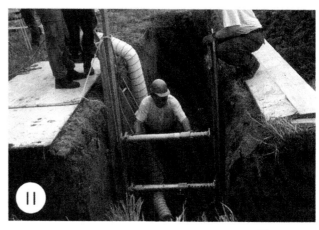

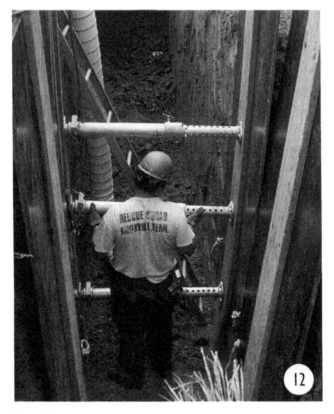

Step 12. Have the crew place another set of panels. ▲

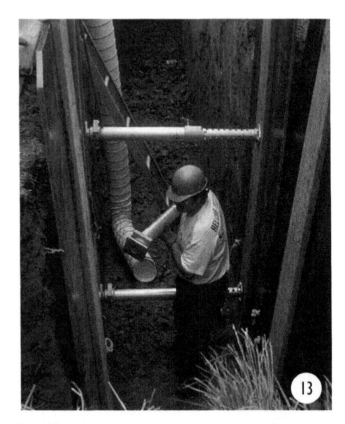

Step 13. Remove the original center shore. ▲

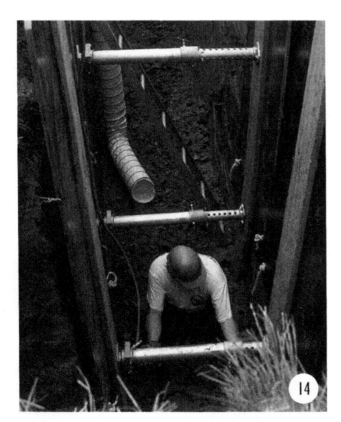

Step 14. Turn and place the center shore on the bottom of the second set of panels. ▲

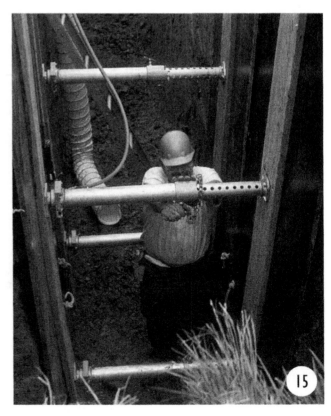

Step 15. Place the top shore. ▲

Step 16. Be sure the corners are square with the top of the "T" trench. ◄

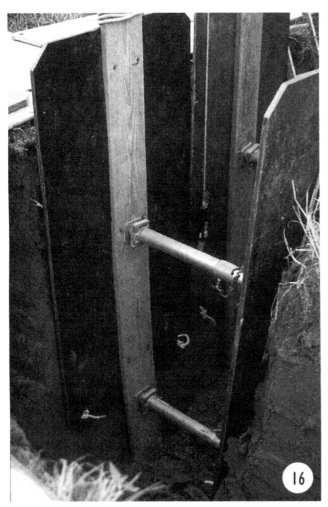

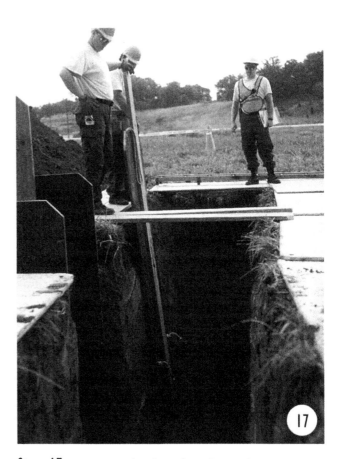

Step 17. Measure back 4 feet from the corner to place the next set of panels. Once again, we are setting up a safety zone to work from. ▲

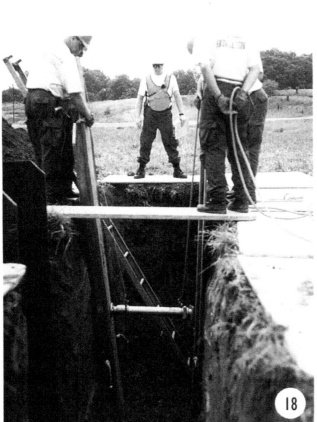

Step 18. Hang and pressurize the center shore. ◄

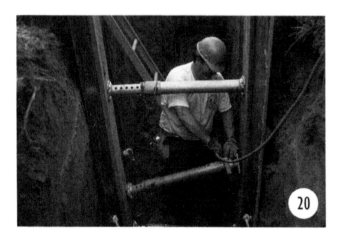

Step 19. Place bottom and top shores.

Step 20. Remove the center shore. ◄

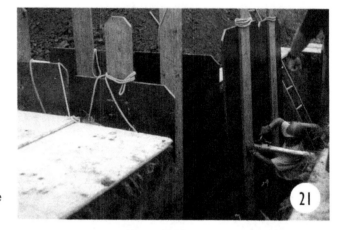

Step 21. Place another set of panels and secure. Note that the corners are butted together. ▶

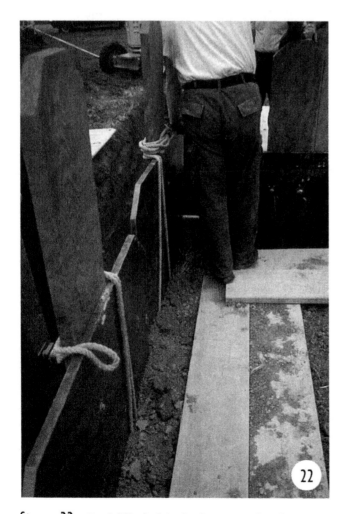

Step 22. Backfill behind the panels, keeping everything tight. ▲

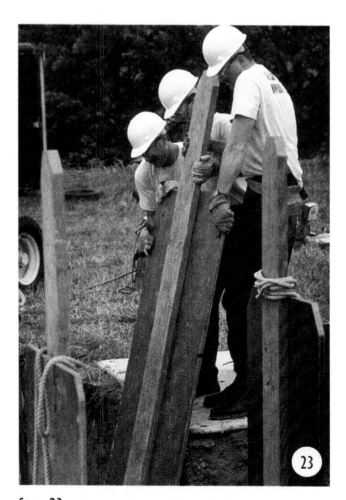

Step 23. Place and shore the identical set of panels on the other side of the "T." ▲

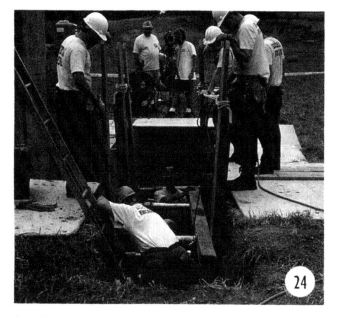

Step 24. Place walers at the top and bottom on the top of the "T" side only. ▲

Step 25. If the open wall of the trench on top of the "T" side is wider than 4 feet, consider dropping a panel behind the wales. If not, use 2-inch by 12-inch by 12-foot planks to seal off the wall. Use wedges to hold the panel or planks in place. ▶

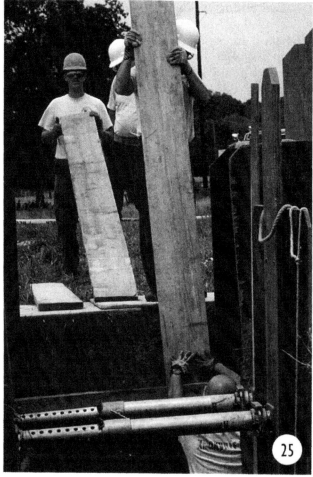

By using walers in this way, you are leaving a vast area in which to work at the top of the "T" without any crossovers. However, if you have to dig any depth (over 2 feet) you must prepare the trench for vertical supplemental sheeting. Or, you can use the horizontal supplemental sheeting that is shown in Phase 8. Either of these methods will work—the choice is yours. The vertical method will add two more wales in the "T." Do not forget your 2- by 12- by 12-inch scabs.

There will be times when it will be desirable to fill in behind the sheeting with air bags as when large sections of the corners are gone. If you choose to undertake this procedure, be extremely careful. Use either medium- or low-pressure bags, because they lend themselves to stuffing behind the sheeting more easily than high-pressure bags. Also, they will conform to the voids in most cases. Inflate them *only to the point of contact.* If they are inflated any further, the sheeting will move in the direction of least resistance, which is upward. Hold your hand on the sheeting. When you feel the slightest movement, shut the system off and disconnect the air line so that there can be no accidental charging of the bags. Check the bags every half-hour for leak-off.

SCENARIO WITH A "T" TRENCH

So far we have explored the methods of safely sheeting and shoring a trench to rescue a victim buried perhaps to the waist (known as a "screamer") or to dig for body recovery. The problems encountered when there is a pipe, boulder, or machine pinning the victim will be discussed in Phase 6—Gaining Access.

At this time, I would like to lead you through one of these scenarios—that of a large-pipe entrapment.

The pipe involved is a 10-foot length of 24-inch concrete storm sewer pipe. It is wire-mesh reinforced and weighs approximately 3000 pounds.

The town fathers decided that the public works department, consisting of four men, would lay a short storm drain line from the highway to a pond. A trench was opened beside the road, 4 feet wide and 8 feet deep, for a distance of 100 feet. At approximately the center of this line, a "T" connection was made to provide a drain to the pond. Because the rubber-tire backhoe being used was light and old, it was used only to dig the trench. The clay walls appeared to be stable—a familiar go-ahead for the foreman—and the foreman chose to ignore the law and not use shoring. Instead, he decided to simply roll the pipe into the trench and draw it together with a light come-along and cement joints.

Everything was progressing smoothly until the crew reached the "T." At that point, the foreman's disregard for safety caught up with them. As they rolled the pipe to the lip of the trench, the corner sheared off and kicked the pipe into the trench at a slight angle. A worker in the trench jumped back, tripped, and fell into a sitting position. The pipe landed on his legs, crushing them, and pinning him against the far wall.

As you arrive on the job site, you are confronted with an unnerving scene: an ancient backhoe, standing up on its rear outriggers, trying its best to lift the pipe. You know it would take an hour to get a crane here from the city, so let's go to work and do the job with the tools at hand.

No one should jump down into the trench to see about the victim until proper sheeting and shoring is complete.

At the scene of a trench accident there can only be one boss. Without reinventing the wheel, you can call that person the "trench boss." This person will make all of the decisions regarding procedures and the overall safety of each person at the trench area. The trench boss should leave issues such as crowd control and medical decisions to the proper authorities; why they would want to get involved in these issues, when the proper personnel have arrived, is beyond me. Once you have delegated this authority, do not pull it back. Of course, you better know your help.

For these reasons, we will not approach the medical aspects of this incident. All I ask is that the trench is not transformed into an emergency room. The trench boss must realize however, that the victim may have crush syndrome and possible spinal injuries.

Step 1. Level all surfaces for ground planks and place the planks.

Step 2. Lay down the ground pads.

Step 3. Monitor the trench for atmospheric conditions.

Step 4. Set up the blower and ventilate the trench.

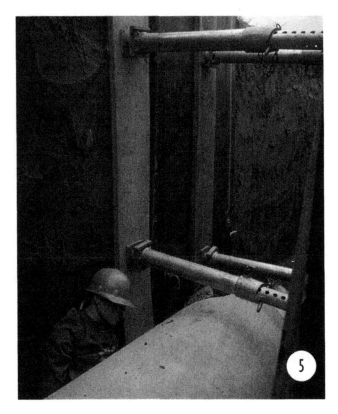

Step 5. Remember that measurements are critical. Place the first set of panels so that they are 4 feet back from the corner and clear of the victim. As you can see, there is room for a 2-inch by 12-inch by 12-foot upright beside the victim. Place a panel opposite and secure shoring to it. Leave space for movement of the pipe. Your medical personnel can now check on the victim's condition. ▲

Step 6. Place a set of panels 4 feet from the top of the "T," providing a safe working area in which to place another set of panels to the corner. ▶

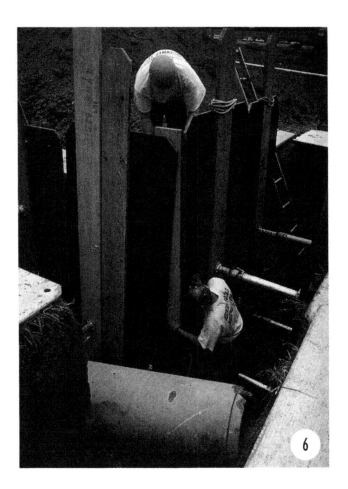

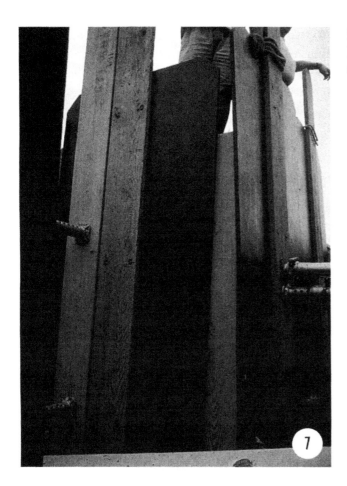

Step 7. Notice the treatment of the corner panels. We have sealed the corner off by inserting an appropriate-sized plank behind the panels. ◄

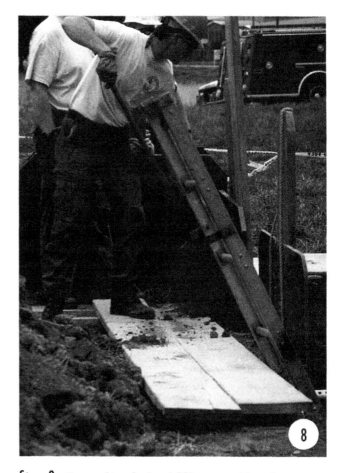

Step 8. Immediately backfill any voids when panels are in place. ▲

Step 9. Finish off the top of the "T" with panels. Be sure they cover the corner on at least one side.

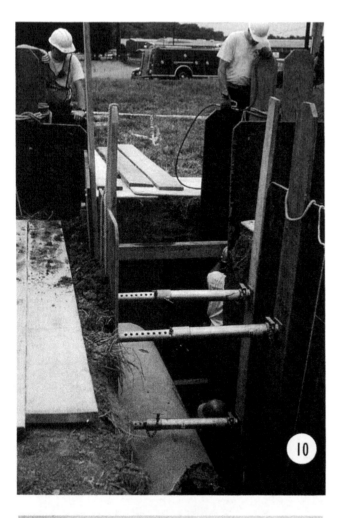

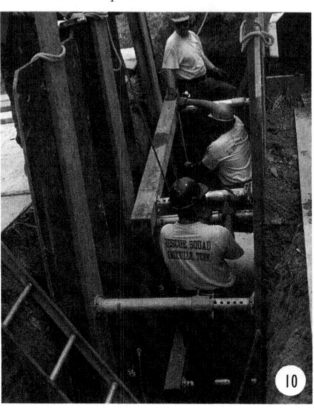

Step 10. Secure the wales in place next. Note that we use them on one side only to hold a panel or uprights and seal off the top of the "T." ◀▼

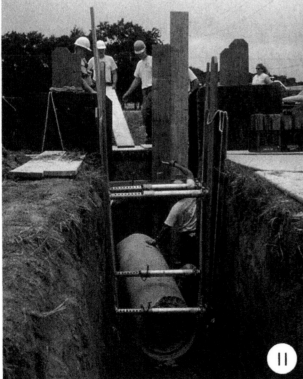

Step 11. Once the wales are in place, drop in the 2-inch by 12-inch by 12-foot uprights. ◀▼

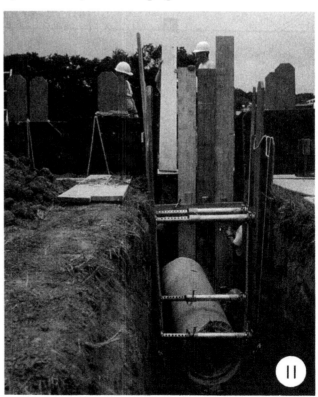

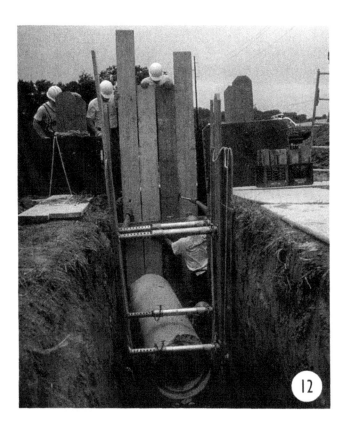

Step 12. Drive wedges between the uprights and the wales, top and bottom. ◄

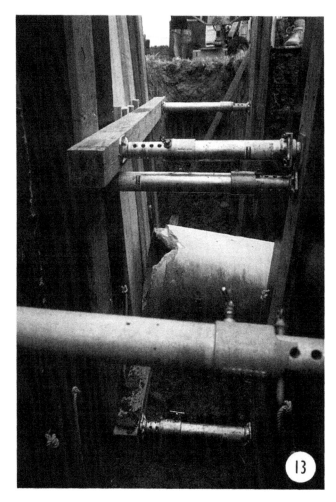

Step 13. The finished job. Note that we went *under* the spigot end of the pipe. It took more effort, but lifting the pipe will be much easier. ▲

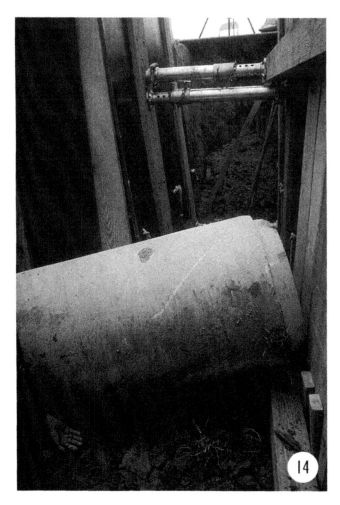

Step 14. A view from the other side shows how close the pipe is to the top of the "T". ◄

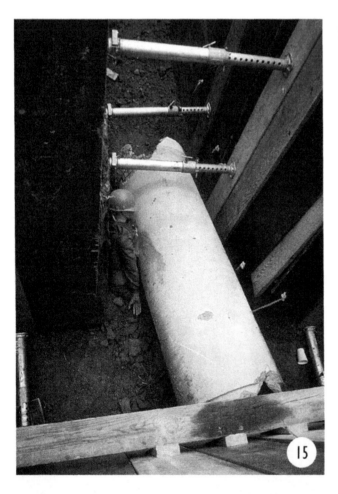

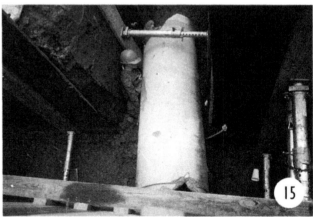

Step 15. At this point, we have to decide if we want to add a shore above the victim's head. We know that we are safe for a horizontal distance of 2 feet from the panel or plank. Since the outside panel is pushing in, it seems best to not add the shore. This will provide more room to extricate the victim. ◀ ▲

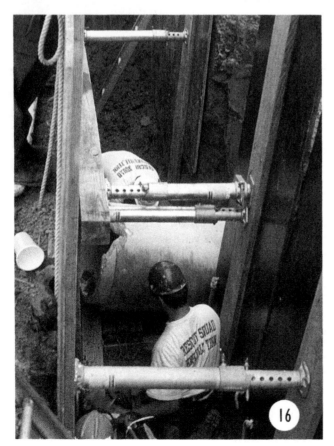

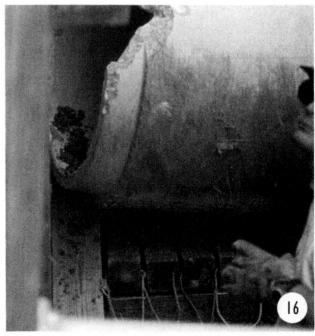

Step 16. Now have the crew place 4- by 4-inch cribbing under the spigot end of the pipe at a slight angle. This will give us a "V" effect under the pipe. ◀ ▲

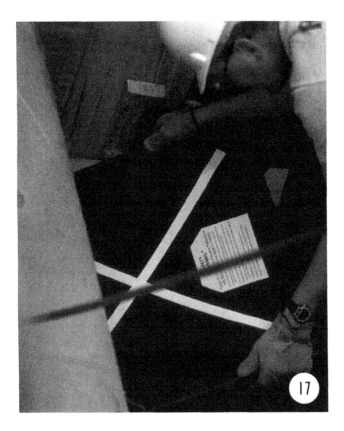

Step 17. Select a matched set of air bags and place them on the cribbing on each side. Slide the bags as far under as you can. To get the proper lift, the bags must be at least halfway under the pipe. ◄

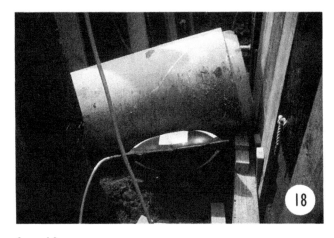

Step 18. Inflate the bags evenly. ▲

Step 19. Be sure you crib under the pipe as you lift. ◄

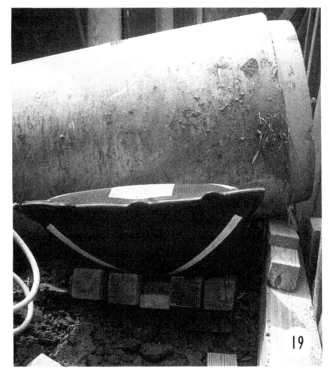

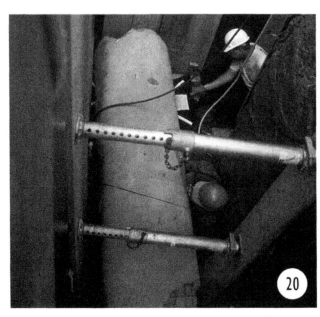

Step 20. The rescuers in the trench must watch the lifting process carefully while keeping an eye on the victim. Lift only high enough to slide the victim out. If you need an inch, lift an inch, *not* 2 inches. ►

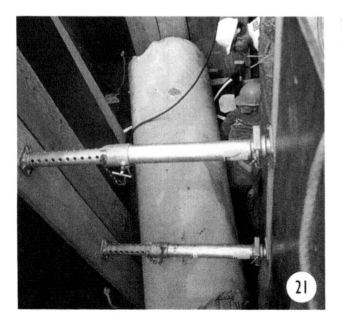

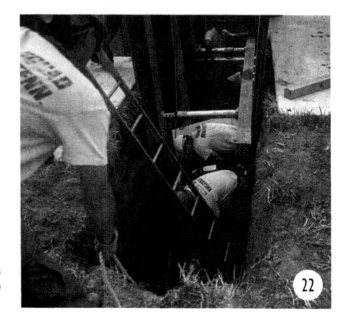

Step 21. When the pipe is lifted high enough, lift and slide the victim out smoothly. ◄

Step 22. Package and remove the victim as quickly as possible; this will be determined by the medics at the scene. ►

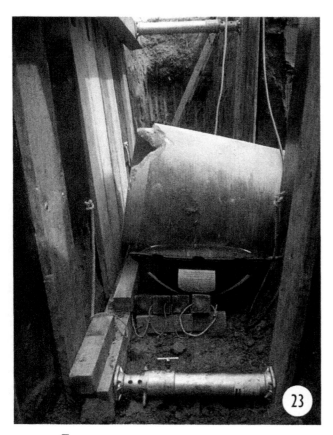

Step 23. Because you have planned your lift, the pipe is free to move on both ends. ◄

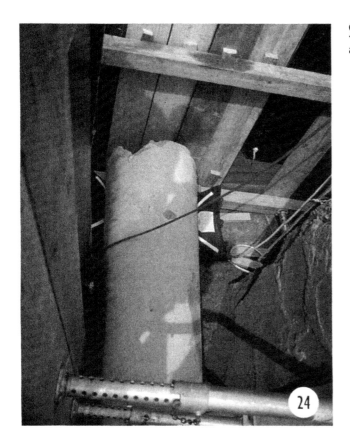

Step 24. Note the tight quarters for the bag placement and the limited space for extricating the victim. ◄

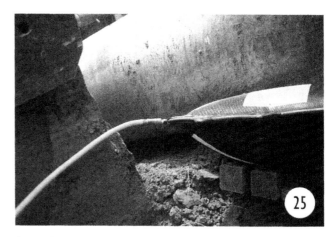

Step 25. As you can see, the total distance the pipe was lifted was less than 6 inches. This is a normal amount for a victim with crushed legs. ▲

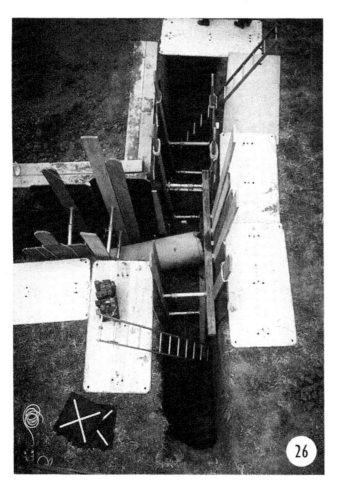

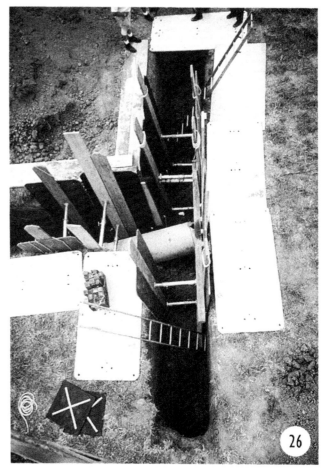

Step 26. Aerial view of the scene, showing the scale of the problem. ▲ ▲

SHORING THE "X" TRENCH

The degree of danger is raised as we move from the "T" to the "X" trench simply because of the additional corners that are liable to break off. The "X" trench is actually a crossover, similar to those found at street intersections when sanitary sewers are installed.

Step 1. Level all surfaces for ground planks.

Step 2. Place the ground planks.

Step 3. Lay down the ground pads.

Step 4. Monitor the trench for atmospheric conditions.

Step 5. Set up the blower and ventilate the trench.

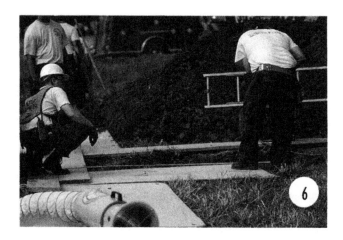

Step 6. The actual steps for sheeting and shoring are similar to the "T" trench, in that you start 4 feet back from the crossover and establish a "safe zone." Once again, measurements are very important. ◄

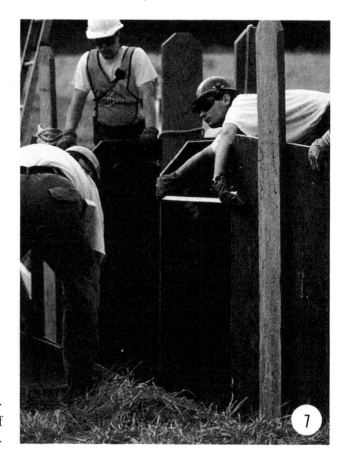

Step 7. If you have measured correctly, the next set of panels will bring you to a point even with the crossover.

Step 8. Repeat this set of panels for each leg of the "X." Resist the temptation to step across and panel from another leg, because the corners are dangerous until covered. This can only be accomplished by working from the "safe zone." ▼ ▶

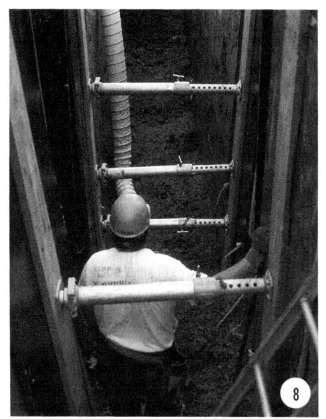

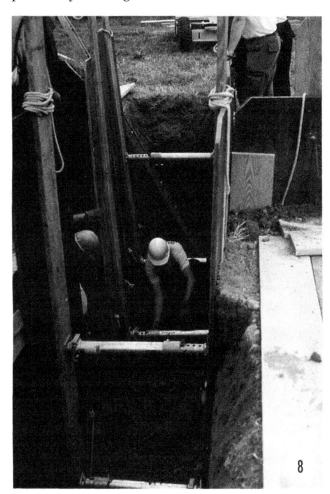

Step 9. The corner where the collapse occurred is particularly troublesome because there is nothing to sheet and shore against. This can be resolved by placing a timber vertically as a strongback. It may take a few timbers. Do not hesitate to fill in behind the sheeting with lumber. ▼ ▶

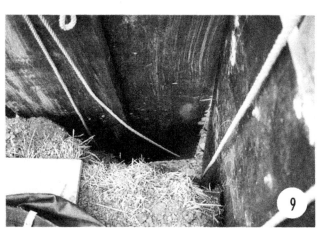

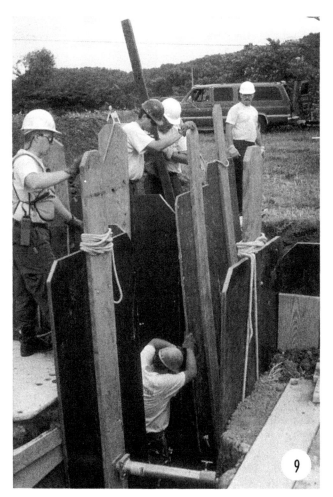

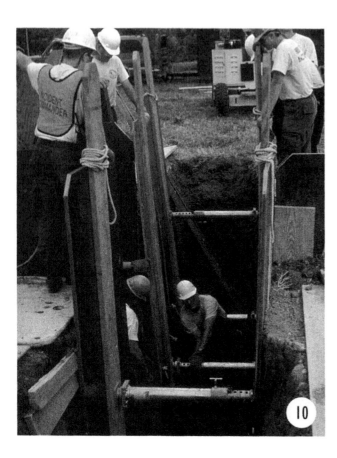

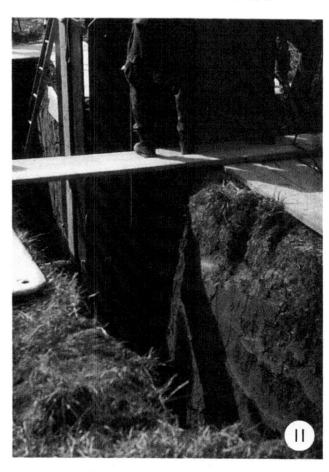

Step 11. Span the trench with planks to make it easier to handle the panels. ►

Step 12. Set up the controls and air supply for low-pressure air bags. ◄

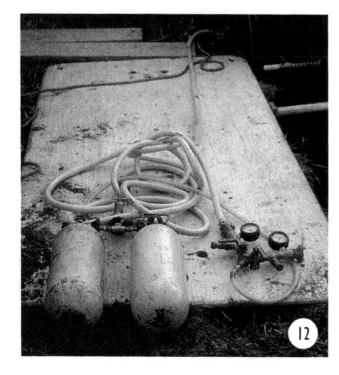

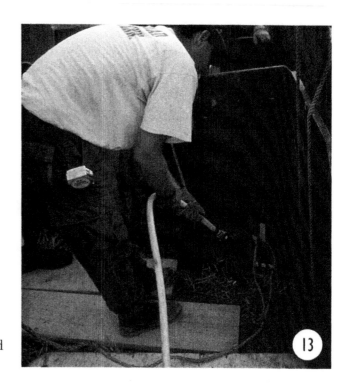

Step 13. Stuff a large low-pressure air bag into the void as far down as you can. ►

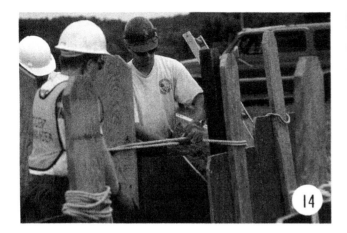 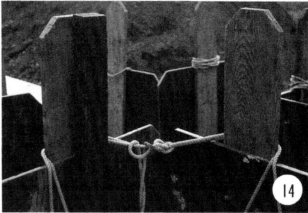

Step 14. Tie the end panels together. ▲ ▲

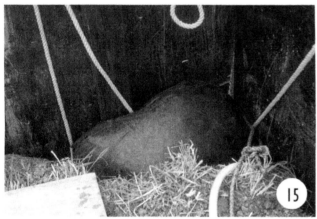 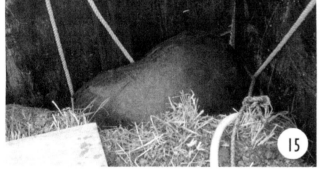

Step 15. Inflate the bag until it makes contact with the panels. Shut the bottles off so that there can be no further pressurization. ◀

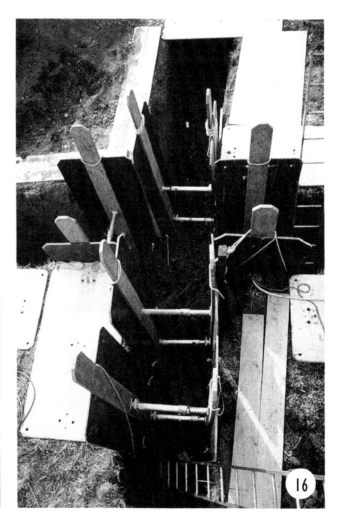

Step 16. Prepare for digging, walers, and supplemental sheeting. ▼ ▶

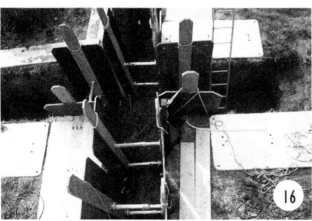

SHORING THE "L" TRENCH

The "L" trench can be said to be the most dangerous trench because the outside corner of the "L" is usually left unshored. If the corner or walls collapse, there is nothing to shore to; so you must create outside wales to span the gaps.

Step 1. Level all surfaces for ground planks.

Step 2. Place the ground planks.

Step 3. Lay down the ground pads.

Step 4. Monitor the trench for atmospheric conditions.

Step 5. Set up the blower and ventilate the trench.

Step 6. Create "safe zones" in both legs of the "L", 4 feet back from the break, and then fill in to the corner. ▶

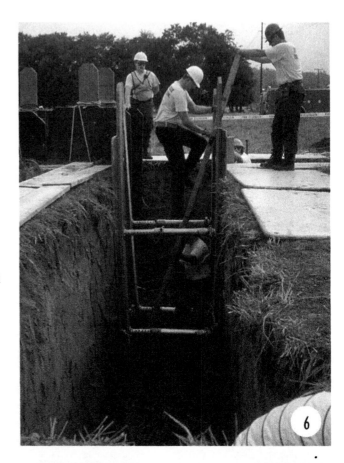

Step 7. While the crew is setting up, have a backhoe operator dig an extension of one leg of the "L", first checking the profile to make sure nothing is underground. This extension should be 4 to 5 feet deep and the same width as the trench. Slope it from the trench up to ground level. If kept under 5 feet, it is not considered a shorable trench. However, for safety's sake, put a shore against two uprights, because you will be kneeling down to assist in placing the wales. ▼ ▶

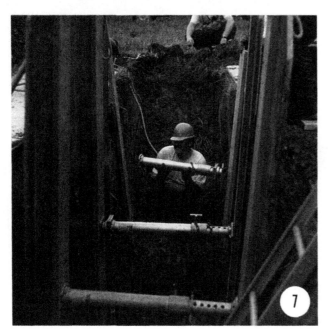

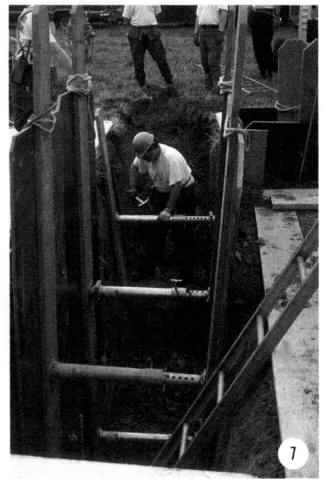

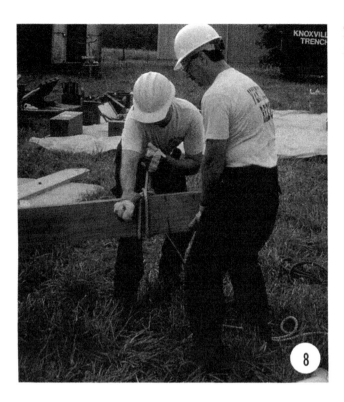

Step 8. All measurements are critical. Wales should remain at 2 feet below the trench lip and be within 4 feet of each other. Notice that we have changed to an 8- by 8-inch wale because the wale must take the side loading in the "L." The ropes on both ends of the wale are for easy handling. ◀

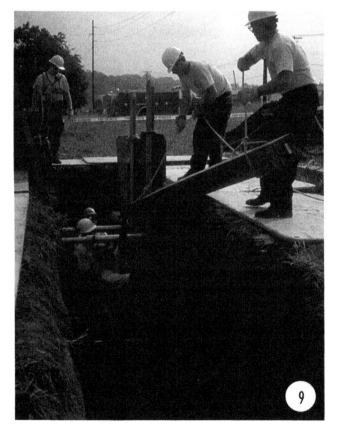

Step 9. Lower the wale into the trench and lay it on top of the bottom shores. Run it all the way through until it touches the headwall in the "L." ◀ ▼

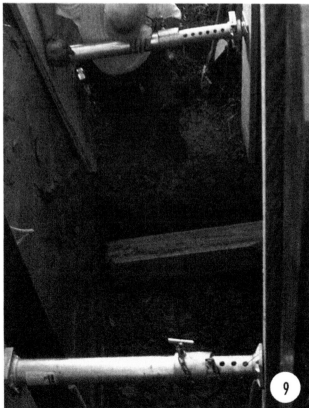

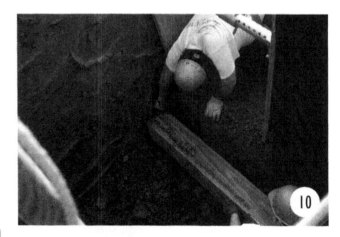

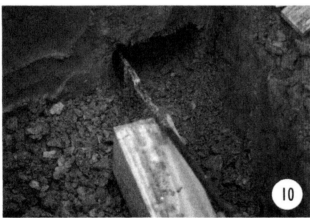

Step 10. Mark the spot where the wale touches the wall. Now lower the wale to the bottom of the trench and cut an 8-inch by 8-inch by 1-foot-deep hole into the wall. If you do not have an air knife, use a post spade and a small shovel. ▲ ◀ ▼

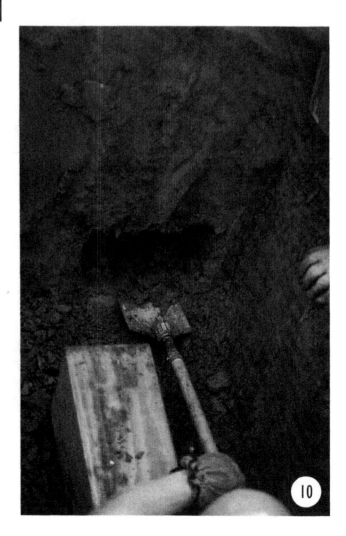

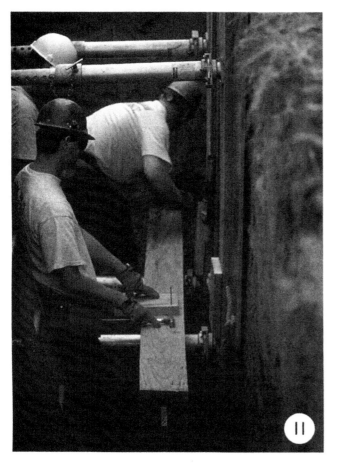

Step 11. While waiting for the hole to be dug, have the crew prepare and nail on 2- by 12- by 12-inch scabs for proper spacing. ◀▼

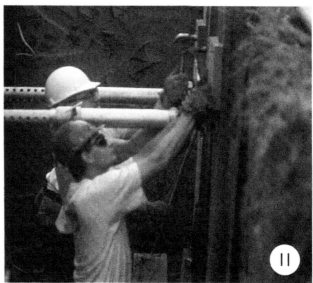

◀

Step 12. Dig the hole 8 to 12 inches deep.

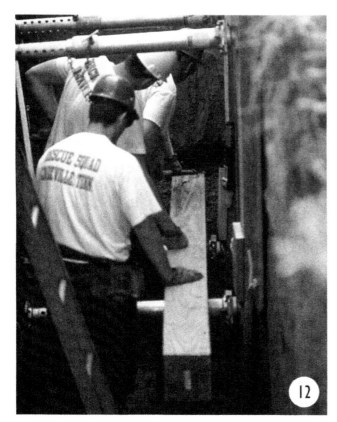

Step 13. Slide the wale all the way into the hole until it bottoms out. ▶

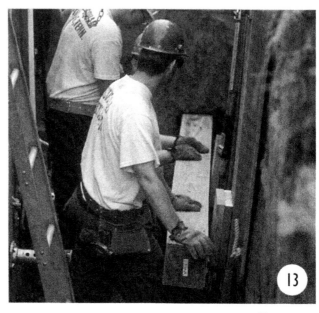

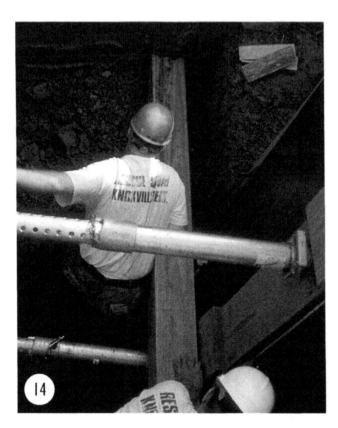

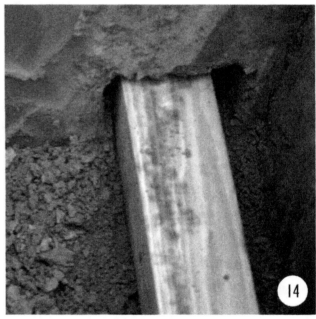

Step 14. Make the hole a few inches larger so as not to bind the wale on the uprights, still keeping the sheeting area fairly tight. ◄ ▼

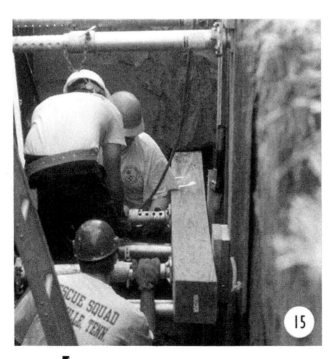

Step 15. Install shores at both uprights. ◄

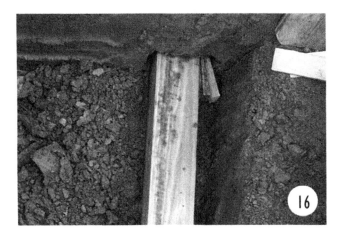

Step 16. Drive wedges into the hole so that the wale cannot move. ◄

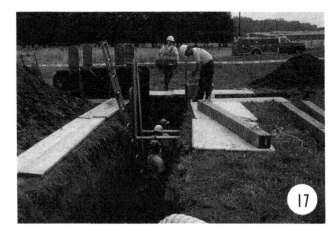

Step 17. Prepare to lower the top wale in place. ►

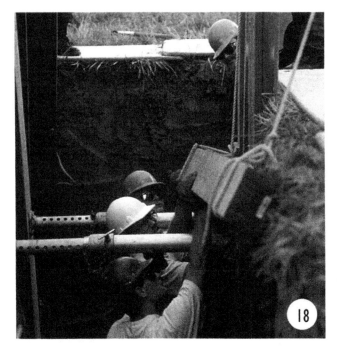

Step 18. Set the wale on the top set of shores. ◄

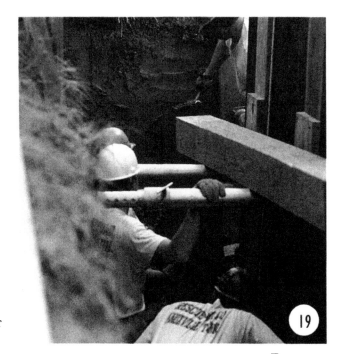

Step 19. Slide the wale forward and mark the wall for cutting the hole. ►

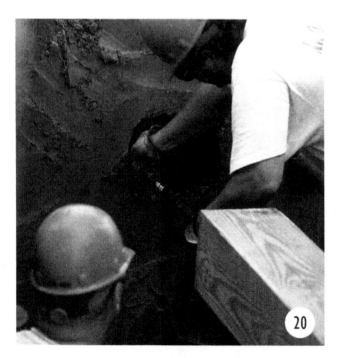

Step 20. Dig a hole 8 to 12 inches deep to accept the wale. ◄ ▼

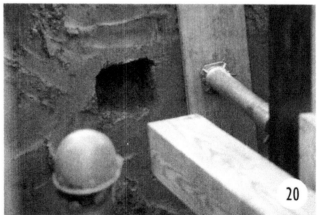

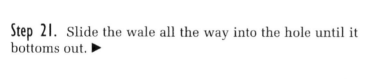

Step 21. Slide the wale all the way into the hole until it bottoms out. ►

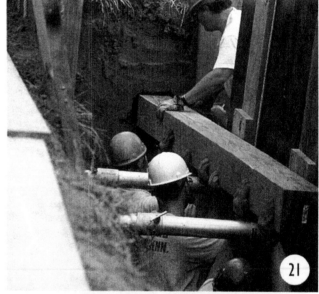

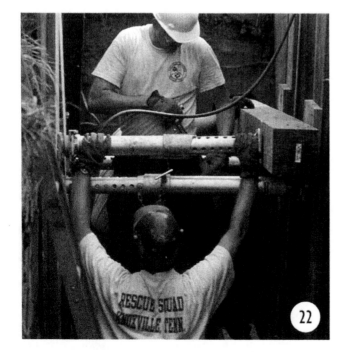

Step 22. Secure the wale on both uprights with shoring. ▲ ►

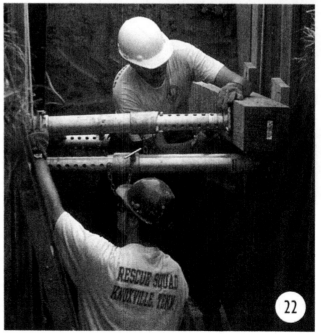

144

Step 23. The following photographs show the trench up to this point:

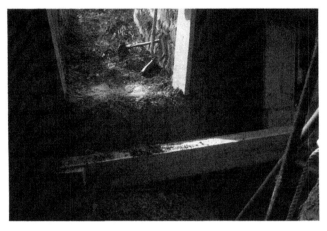

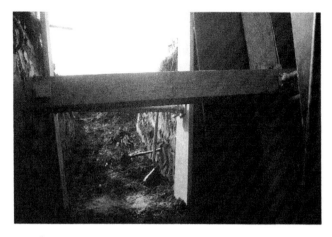

- The bottom wale embedded in the wall at the top of the "L," looking into the 5-foot trench.

- The same view, showing the top wale.

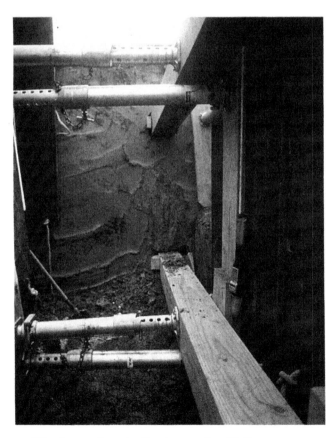

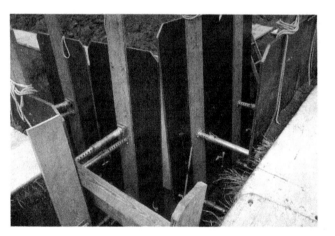

- The top view of the "L" trench.

- The long view to the top or the "L."

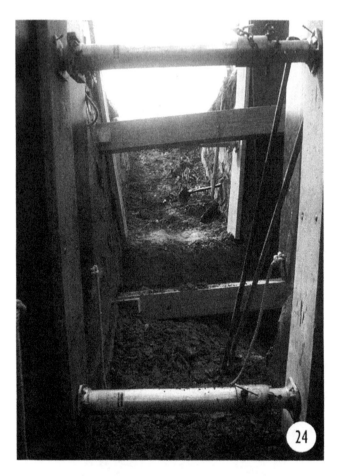

Step 24. Prepare now for the other leg of the "L." ◄

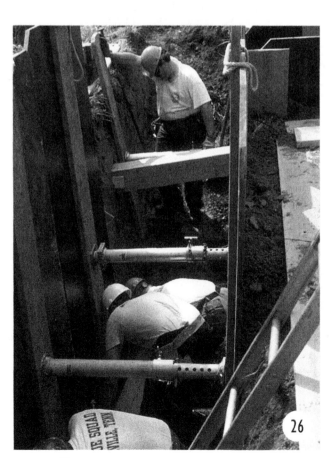

Step 25. Bring another 8-inch by 8-inch by 12-foot timber around to the side of the trench. ▲

Step 26. Lower it to the bottom and place it on the bottom shores. ◄

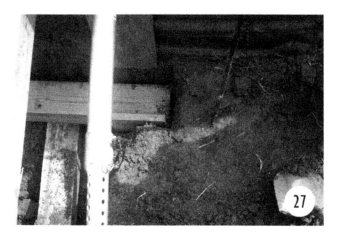

Step 27. Dig a slit in the short trench and slide the wale over the other bottom wale. ◄

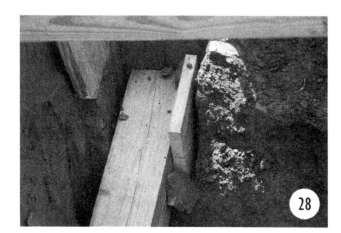

Step 28. Fill in any gap with lumber. ▶

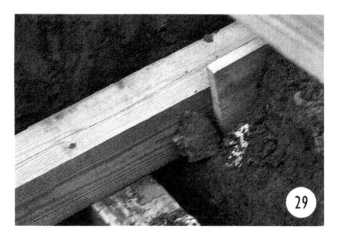

Step 29. Note the perfect fit of the wales; one supports the other. ◄

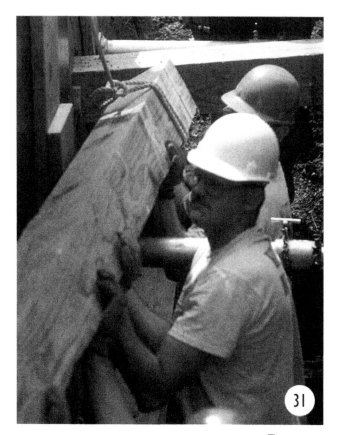

Step 30. Secure the bottom wale with shoring.

Step 31. Place the top wale. ▶

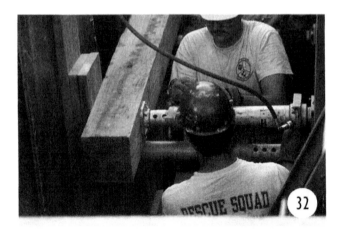

Step 32. Secure the back end. ◀

Step 33. Place any fillers needed. ▶

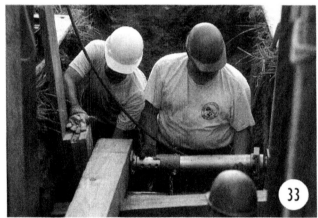

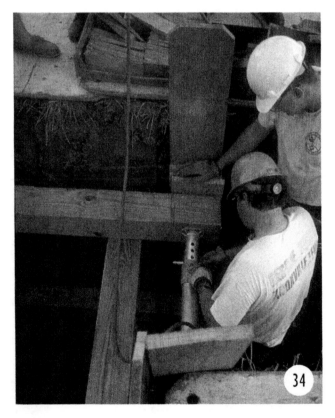

Step 34. Secure the "L" end. ◀

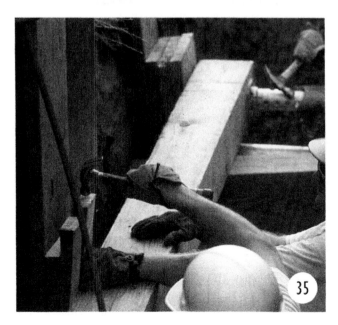

Step 35. Drive wedges in any gaps. ▶

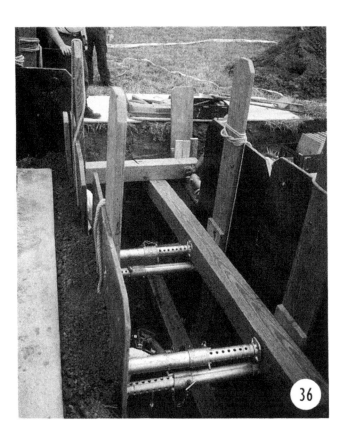

Step 36. The wales are now finished and are awaiting 2-inch by 12-inch by 12-foot uprights for sheeting. ◄

Step 37. Place uprights. ▲

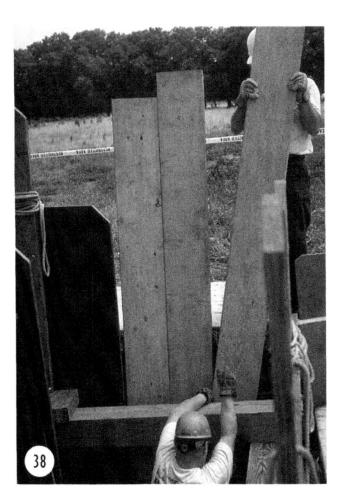

◄
Step 38. Run the uprights all the way across tightly. If the trench were wide enough for a 4-foot panel, we could use it here.

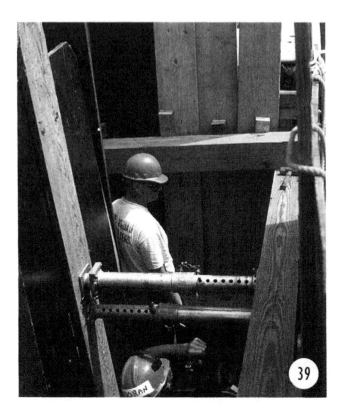

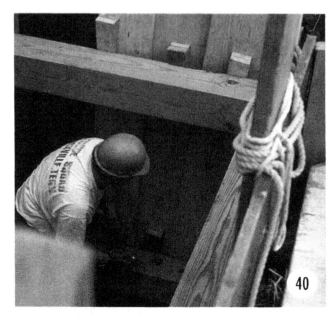

Step 39. Wedge all the uprights across the top. ◄

Step 40. Then wedge all the uprights across the bottom. ▲

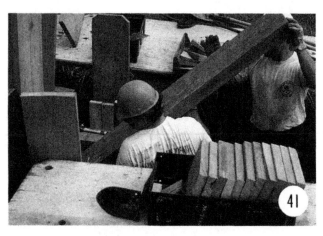

Step 41. Before placing the uprights on the short trench side, install a 4-inch by 4-foot timber on a diagonal between the wale and the double shoring. This will fill in the gap so that the wedges will take up the rest. There will be very little pressure on the top part of the uprights, so side-loading the shores is not a problem. ▲

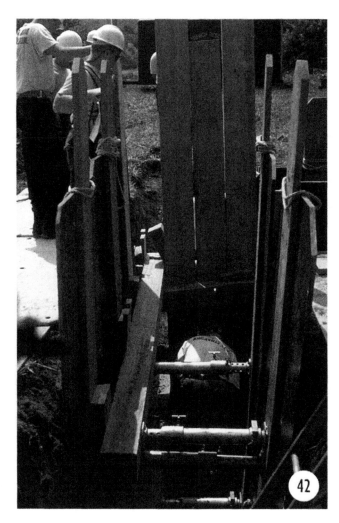

Step 42. Now fill in with uprights. ►

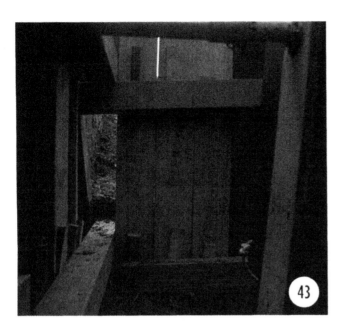

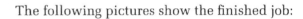

Step 43. Wedge the uprights top and bottom. ◀

The following pictures show the finished job:

- Outside the short trench, showing the diagonal timber.

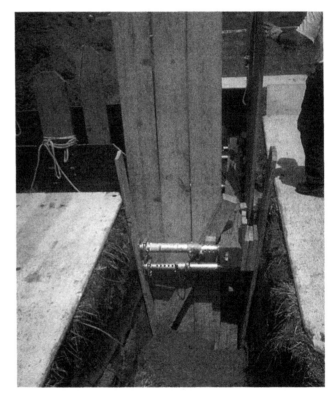

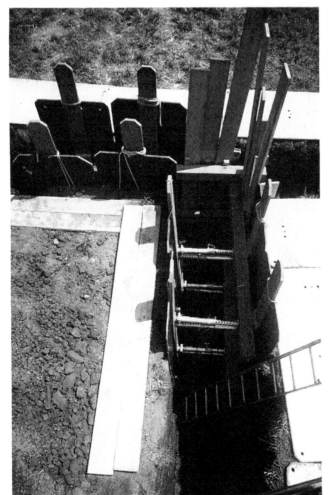

- Aerial view.

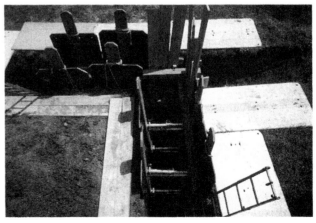

SHORING THE HAND-DUG WELL

In the early years of our country, hand-dug wells were in demand to supply water for both domestic and commercial purposes. As gridiron systems were installed, these wells were filled in or covered over. Many of these wells are being rejuvenated for domestic purposes, and occasionally someone falls through the cover cap.

These wells are generally 4 to 6 feet in diameter and 30 to 40 feet deep. Some are brick- or fieldstone-lined, but many are not lined at all. The very fact that they are round in most cases prevents cave-ins, because the soil supports itself. The main danger is loss of life from asphyxiation, generally when a crew goes into a well to clean it out. A well is a confined space and must be treated as such.

If you are dispatched for rescue in such an incident, determine whether the well is lined or unlined. A good light will help to determine if the lining is intact or crumbling. If the latter is true, or if the well us unlined, you should treat the well as you would an unshored trench.

Step 1. Place ground pads all the way around the opening.

Step 2. Monitor the well for atmospheric conditions.

Step 3. Have crew members who will be working near the well put on full body harnesses and lifelines rigged to the rear "D" ring. Determine anchor points for the lifelines. Keep the anchor points spaced so as to prevent tangling.

Step 4. Set up the blower and ventilate the well.

Step 5. Rig an ascent/descent device to a tripod, A-frame, wrecker, crane, or any other means that can be used as an anchor point 10 feet above the ground level. *Do not* use any motor-driven retrieval system.

Step 6. Nail scabs on two 2-inch by 8-inch, 10-inch, or 12-inch by 12-foot planks at $1\frac{1}{2}$-foot, $5\frac{1}{2}$-foot, and $9\frac{1}{2}$ foot spacings and 2-foot, 6-foot, and 10-foot spacings on two more planks.

Step 7. Suspend the evenly spaced planks in the well across from each other and install your shoring on the top scabs. (If you are using pneumatic shoring, there is no need for scabs.)

Step 8. Suspend the unevenly spaced planks in the well at a 90-degree angle to those already installed. Place the shores from the top down.

Step 9. Lower the rescuer(s) into the well, installing shoring as they go down.

Step 10. Add uprights and shoring to the bottom.

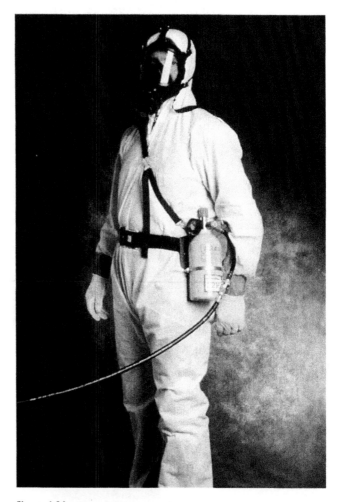

Figure 4-20. Supplied air systems.

> **Note**
> Because this is a confined-space exercise, we recommend the use of supplied-air systems for the rescuer(s). (Figure 4-20).

Remember that the situations just discussed are the ones that you are most likely to encounter in trenches up to 12 feet deep. Become familiar with the techniques of sheeting and shoring for these "standard" situations. Then when you are faced with more unusual circumstances, you will be able to adapt. Remember, also, that you should not attempt to sheet and shore a trench that is deeper than 15 feet; the danger is too great.

You may wonder, then, what you can do with a trench that is between 12 and 15 feet deep. Making safe a trench that is 15 feet deep involves installing prefabricated sheeting both vertically and horizontally. Figure 4-21 shows a 15-foot trench that has been properly sheeted and shored.

Shoring is accomplished from the top down. The vertical panels are lowered to the bottom of the trench with ropes. While rescuers hold the vertical panels in place and prevent them from slipping sideways, other rescuers install the horizontal panels. Once the horizontal panels are shored in place, the lower panels are shored from the top down.

Keep in mind that the size of timber shores should be relative to the width and depth of the trench. Refer to the OSHA chart to see what size timbers should be used for trenches up to 15 feet deep.

ALTERNATIVE TECHNIQUES FOR MAKING A TRENCH SAFE

Undoubtedly the question has come to mind: "What can I use to make a trench safe when there just aren't any of the conventional sheeting and shoring materials available?"

There are two items that often are found at underground utility construction sites: trench boxes and precast concrete structures. Both can be used for the protection of victims and rescuers alike during trench rescue operations.

USING A TRENCH BOX

Utility contractors throughout the country use trench boxes (often called trench shields) when they are faced with the problems of hydrostatic conditions in the soil, sand, and bad ground.

Trench boxes are usually made of steel and aluminum. They range in size from 6 feet high by 16 feet long to 8 feet by 20 feet, although custom-made boxes may exceed these dimensions. The width of a trench box can be varied by means of spreaders made of pipe, steel beams, and, in the cast of larger boxes, steel arches. Trench boxes weigh from 3100 pounds to more than 12,000 pounds, depending on the size and the material used (Figure 4-22).

A trench box provides a safe working area for a pipe-laying crew. Once the trench is dug, the box is

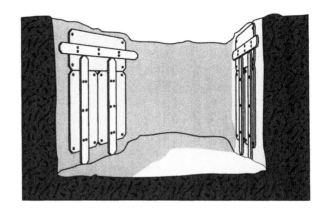

Figure 4-21. A properly sheeted and shored trench.

lowered into the trench or dragged into place with a backhoe. It is moved with the backhoe as the pipe-laying progresses.

Trench boxes are similar to conventional sheeting and shoring devices in one respect: they are often found at the side of the job site—not in place where they should be—when the foreman has decided that speed is more important than safety.

If you arrive on the scene of a trench accident without sheeting and shoring materials and without the prospect of obtaining any from community resources,but there is a trench box at hand, use this technique for making the trench safe when the victim is completely buried.

> **Remember**
> It is not advisable to use the same operator who was running the backhoe at the time of the incident. Your community resource list should provide names of contractors previously contacted who can supply operators.

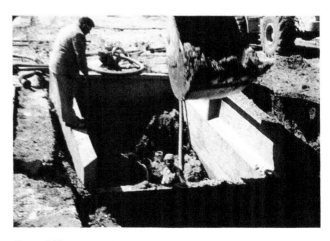

Figure 4-22. A trench box.

1. Establish the centerline of the original trench if there has been a massive cave-in.
2. Mark the perimeter of the trench. This line will guide the backhoe operator.
3. Determine the approximate location of the victim from available clues.
4. Have the backhoe operator lift the box and center it above the suspected location of the victim.
5. If the trench is deeper than the box is high, have the operator slope the portions of the wall that tower over the box. Be sure to have at least 18 inches of the box exposed.
6. Place a ladder in the box. Have the rescue crew enter the box after monitoring the atmosphere and ventilating. Start the digging operations.
7. Each time the rescuers remove a foot of spoil from the box, have the operator press the box deeper into the trench. Instruct him to press the side walls of the box with his bucket. Caution him against trying to "hammer" the box down by striking its sides with the bucket. The lower

edges of the box sides are provided with knife edges; thus the box can be sunk into the trench floor with little effort. By having rescuers remove a foot of dirt at a time, you will be able to see that the victim's limbs are not under the knife edges before the box is pushed down.

8. Have the rescuers dig until they uncover the victim. See that they keep the bottom of the trench level as they dig.

ALUMINUM TRENCH BOX

The newest innovation on the market is an aluminum trench box weighing less than 1000 pounds, which is designed for 16 feet in class "C" soil. Built for the contractor making repairs, this box is ideal for rescuers. It can be carried in pieces and assembled in 15 minutes. Because rescue crews can use the pneumatic struts they already own, the box can handle trenches 3 to 12 feet wide. The box shown is 6 by 10 feet, with supplemental panels of 2 by 10 feet. It can be used horizontally or vertically and is available in many different sizes, up to 12 feet long.

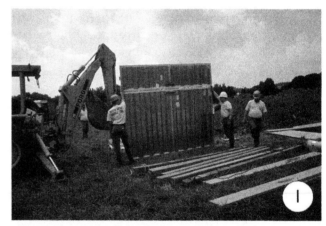

INSTALLING THE ALUMINUM TRENCH BOX

Step 1. The box sides and components are first laid out on the ground. ▼ ▶

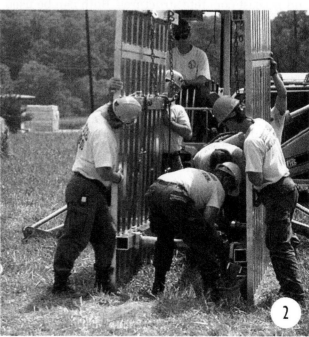

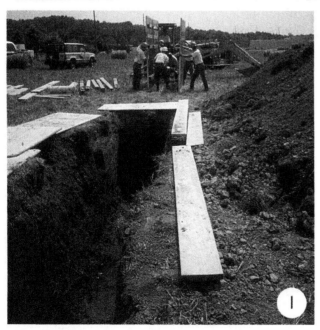

Step 2. After putting the slide brackets in place, stand the sides vertically. ▶

Step 3. Connect pneumatic struts to the slide brackets. ◄

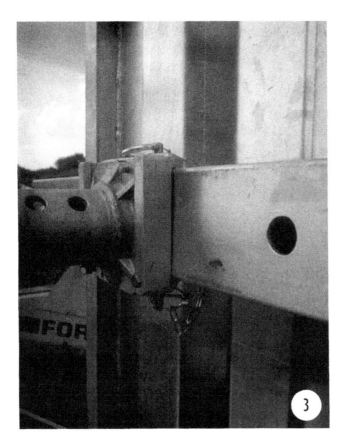

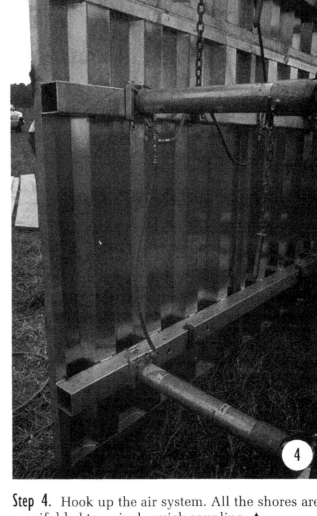

Step 4. Hook up the air system. All the shores are manifolded to a single quick coupling. ▲

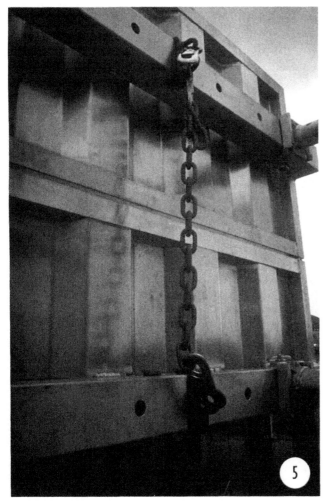

◄

Step 5. The 2- by 10-foot supplemental panels can be placed on top of the box by pins in the end and chains, as shown, or they can be added every 2 feet on the bottom, or both. By placing additional panels after digging 2 feet, you need only to pass the panels in and pressurize the shores on both ends. Note the waler built into the supplemental panel. This replaces the vertical or horizontal planking needed for supplemental sheeting.

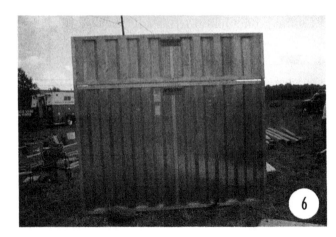

Step 6. Completely assemble the box.
◄

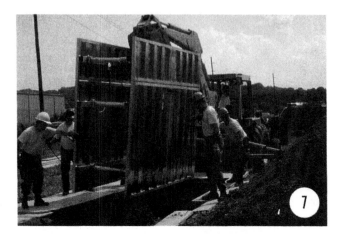

Step 7. Lift the box by a wire rope bridle. ▶

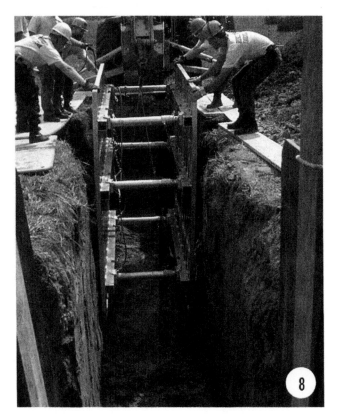

Step 8. Place the box in the trench. If for any reason a lifting device is not available, the rescue crew could pull the box into the trench by tying ropes on the bottom shores and dragging it.
◄

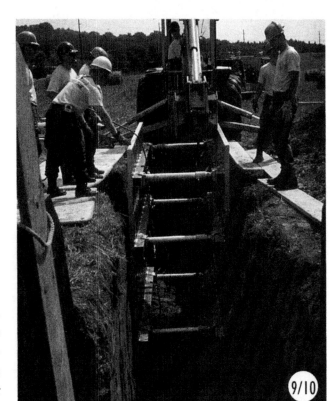

Step 9. The box should be placed directly over a live victim, or in the approximate location of a buried body.

Step 10. Pressurize the shores at a recommended 200 psi, which is the same pressure you have been using for the struts. ▶

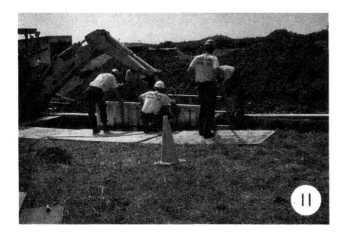

Step 11. Place a ladder in the trench and monitor the atmosphere. ◄

Step 12. Have a rescuer descend and pin out all the shores. ►

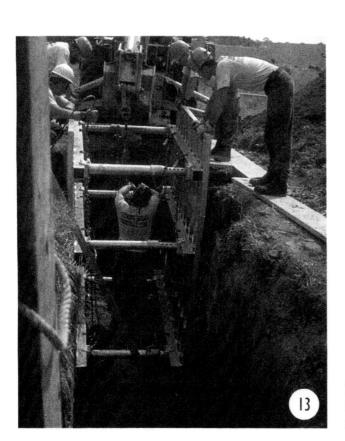

Step 13. The supplemental panels are not manifolded into the rest of the system. Pin and lock them out separately. ◄

157

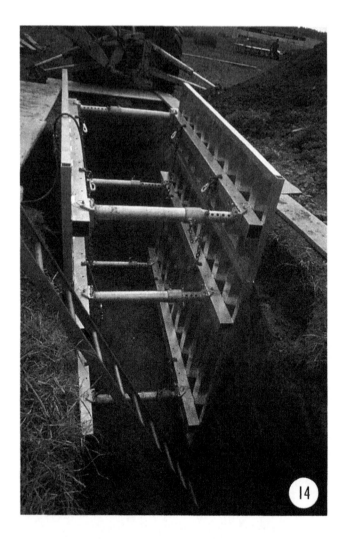

◄▼
Step 14. Connect the blower and ventilate the trench. Shown are views of the finished box from both ends.

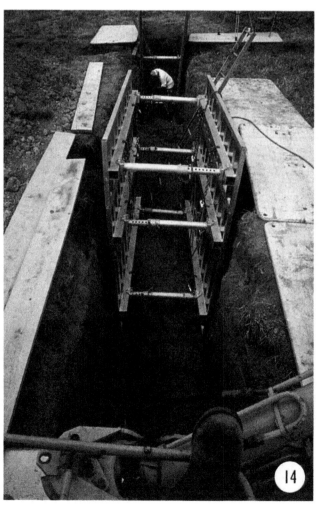

USING PRECAST CONCRETE STRUCTURES

Precast concrete manhole rings, precast concrete catch basins, and even precast concrete electrical vault sections can be used to protect a trench-accident victim who is only partially buried (Figure 4-23). The structure is positioned so that it surrounds the victim while the trench walls are cut back to the angle of repose. Needless to say, there must be enough room for the casting between the trench wall and the victim.

Precast concrete manhole rings are generally 48 inches in diameter and from 3 to 4 feet deep. Precast catch basins and electrical vault sections are usually larger; some measure as much as 8 by 12 feet.

Consider using this technique when you have only a precast manhole ring available for protecting a partially covered victim during a trench rescue operation. Because the heavy concrete structure must be swung directly over the victim and then lowered until it surrounds him, it is imperative that the crane or backhoe operator be a calm, cool individual with a steady hand on the controls. I certainly suggest that you do not use the operator who was working at the time of the accident and who was possibly even responsible for the mishap.

1. Locate the gear that is used for lifting and lowering the manhole section. This will be a two-, three-, or four-leg wire rope or chain bridle that has the legs joined with a steel ring or oval. There will be dowel pins at the end of each leg. You should be able to find this rigging next to the manhole, in a workman's pickup truck, or in the tool trailer. If you cannot find the rigging, ask someone. It is vital to the operation.
2. Most backhoes have a large slip hook welded to the back of the bucket to facilitate lifting heavy objects. Have the operator curl the bucket. Place the ring or oval of the lifting bridle in the throat of the hook. If there is no such hook, secure the bridle to the bucket with a wire rope and shackle or a chain that is provided with grab hooks. Do not catch the ring or oval of the lifting bridle with a bucket tooth; it could fall off and cause the manhole section to fall when it is over the victim.
3. Place the dowel pins of the lifting rig in the holes provided in the concrete casting.
4. Have the operator lift the casting. Check the rigging. Have a competent signalman work with the operator so that commands can be relayed correctly.
5. Have the operator boom the casting over the trench slowly so that there is minimal swinging. When the casting is still, have the operator lower it gently over the victim. Be careful that the ladder that is built into the interior wall of the

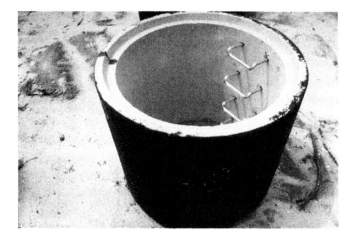

Figure 4-23. A pre-cast manhole ring.

casting does not contact the victim. It will be wise to have a workman ride the casting and direct the operator. He will be able to look down into the casting and ensure the victim's safety.

6. Have the workman disconnect the rigging from the backhoe.
7. Instruct the backhoe operator to cut the trench walls back to the angle of repose.
8. When the trench walls are cut back, have the workman reconnect the lifting bridle to the backhoe hook.
9. Instruct the backhoe operator to lift the casting from around the victim.
10. Have the rescuers continue with the digging effort.

If a crane is available at the job site, use it for moving the manhole ring. Valuable time can be saved if you do not have to unrig the backhoe for use in cutting back the trench walls, and then rerig it for lifting the casting.

USING MAKESHIFT MATERIALS FOR SHEETING AND SHORING

I firmly believe that conventional sheeting and shoring materials should be used during a trench rescue effort, and I will argue that virtually every fire department and rescue squad can find the proper materials somewhere in their service areas. Nonetheless, I would be remiss if I did not at least mention items that can be used to form makeshift sheeting and shoring when nothing else is available.

ITEMS THAT CAN BE USED AS UPRIGHTS

Fire department ladders. Fire department–quality ladders can be effectively used as wales or uprights. Do not impose shores directly against the ladder rungs, however. Instead, make rigid foundations for the shores from sections of 2-inch plank and be sure that the planks are long enough to span at least three rungs. Secure the planks to the ladder rungs by driving long nails at the ends of the planks, mating them to the ladder, and bending the nails over the rungs. You can use wall ladders as uprights. However, use only two- or three-section extension ladders for walers, because the side-loading over a distance is far more severe.

Highway guardrails. Steel or aluminum guardrails are very strong, not only because of the material used but also because of the manner in which they are stamped. They make good uprights, but the waves that give them strength also make it difficult to hold shores fast against them. It is suggested that you cut the shores a bit larger than necessary if you are using timbers. You will have to drive them in place with a maul, and when so driven there will be less of a chance for them to slip. Remember that you will not be able to nail the shores to the uprights in the usual manner.

Steel curb forms. Like guardrails, curb forms are very strong. The suggestions made earlier for seating timber shores against guardrails apply here.

ITEMS THAT CAN BE USED FOR SHEETING
Steel concrete forms. Concrete forms are excellent for solid sheeting operations; however, they are heavy and somewhat difficult to handle. If you choose to use steel forms, face them with 2- by 12-inch plank uprights so that the shores can be installed securely. Cut timber shores a bit larger than necessary so that they will hold the uprights rigidly against the forms when they are forced into position.

Solid core doors. Solid core doors are usually strong, but their lack of substantial width may present a problem. Shores will have to be installed on 30- to 36-inch centers, depending on the width of the doors. Their being so close together may seriously hinder the digging and victim-removal operations.

Steel scaffolding. Although scaffolding is nothing more than a framework of steel pipes, sections of scaffolding may adequately support fairly compact trench walls when the sections are held in place with suitable shores. Once again, the use of 2- by 12-inch plank uprights is essential.

ITEMS THAT CAN BE USED FOR SHORING
Tree sections. Tree limbs and trunks are often found piled on construction sites, the result of land-clearing operations. If you have nothing else to use for shoring, cut straight sections of limbs and trunks at least 6 inches in diameter. Cut the sections slightly larger than necessary so that they will have to be driven into place against the uprights and sheeting.

Steel pipe. Steel pipe is used with screw jacks. Sections of steel pipe at least 2-inches in diameter

can also be used alone as makeshift shores. A problem is that the pipe sections have to be cut precisely so that they can be wedged in place. They do not provide the adjustment feature offered by screw jacks. Keep in mind that the maximum length for 2-inch pipe shores is 5 feet.

The Jimmi Jak® rescue tool. Jimmi Jaks® follow the principle and construction features of pneumatic shores, and they will support the same load. However, a squad carrying Jimmi Jaks® will have only four available, and two of the four jacks may be too small to be effective (Figure 4-24).

There are undoubtedly other items that can be pressed into service as makeshift sheeting and shoring devices. Take care in selecting them. The use of materials such as thin sheets of plywood or particle board, backboards or sheets of dry wall, or hollow core doors is not recommended for sheeting. Avoid using pieces of small-diameter pipe, sections of 2- by 4-inch lumber, lengths of plastic pipe, and smoke ejector hangers as shoring. You may spend considerable time on the sheeting and shoring effort and end up with no more protection that the trench walls would offer if they were left unsupported.

A FINAL IMPORTANT POINT
All of the techniques for installing conventional sheeting and shoring were designed first of all with safety in mind. At no time are rescuers required to work in unsupported (thus unsafe) areas. This may not be the case when it is necessary to use makeshift devices. If you cannot lower shores in place with ropes, for example, rescuers may have to make initial installations in a less-than-safe environment. Regardless of what you use in a makeshift operation, and regardless of how much you are motivated to make a quick rescue, be careful! Take no unnecessary chances. Use accepted safe practices whenever you can, and create new safe practices when it appears that you cannot make a trench safe "by the book."

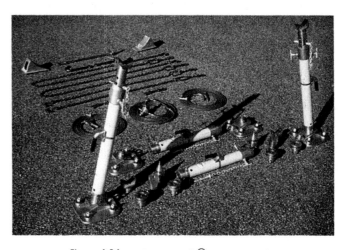

Figure 4-24. A Jimmi Jak® rescue tool.

THE PARKWAY INCIDENT—
HAZARD CONTROL

During the assessment phase of the operation, you looked for hazards that might interfere with the rescue effort. Now, how would you handle some of those hazards?

What would you do about traffic? _____
_____
_____

Who would you assign to the task of traffic control? _____
_____
_____

    On the rescue site plan, indicate with these symbols, -X-X-X-X-, where you would establish the perimeter line for spectators.

Suppose that there were downed electric wires blocking access to the trench area. What would you do?
_____
_____

Suppose that you were faced with a broken water service line in the trench. What would you do?
_____
_____

    Let's say that there is a deep-well system dewatering the ground around the trench, and that the pumps are being operated by a 660-volt electrical source. What would happen if the power source failed. Would you be able to provide a 660-volt supply?

If not, where would you be able to get one? _____
_____
_____

    Now let's see what you would do with other hazards. On the rescue site plan, indicate with symbols and legends where you would position:

- A FRESH-AIR BLOWER
- 2- BY 12-INCH GROUND PLANKS
- 4- BY 8-FOOT GROUND PADS
- THE SAFETY OBSERVER

You are now ready to make the trench safe. In the space below, list the steps for installing the sheeting and shoring that you have available. Try to list them from memory; then when you are finished, read through the text again to see how well you did.

_____

_____

_____

_____

_____

_____

Support Operations

KNOWLEDGE OBJECTIVES

The rescuer should be able to—

- ☑ Define relevant words and phrases
- ☑ Summarize activities of the support phase of a trench rescue operation
- ☑ Describe the procedure for locating and establishing a command post
- ☑ List the contents of a command post kit
- ☑ Describe the need and procedure for creating a parking area for nonessential vehicles
- ☑ Describe the need and procedure for creating a staging area for essential vehicles
- ☑ Describe the need and procedure for creating a supply point
- ☑ Relate the need for continuing traffic and spectator control measures
- ☑ Describe procedures for lighting the scene
- ☑ Relate the importance of keeping the ventilating system operating throughout the rescue effort
- ☑ Describe procedures for protecting the trench from rain, sleet, and snow
- ☑ Describe procedures for rotating and refreshing personnel during the rescue effort
- ☑ Describe activities designed to support family members
- ☑ Describe procedures for cooperating with news media personnel

SKILLS OBJECTIVES

The rescuer working individually or as part of a team should be able to—

- ☑ Establish a command post
- ☑ Make up a command post kit
- ☑ Locate and establish a parking area for nonessential vehicles
- ☑ Locate and establish a staging area for essential vehicles
- ☑ Locate and establish a supply point
- ☑ Manage traffic and spectators
- ☑ Continue contractor-initiated dewatering operations
- ☑ Light the scene
- ☑ Keep ventilating systems operating
- ☑ Protect the trench from rain, sleet, and snow
- ☑ Rotate and refresh rescue personnel
- ☑ Support the needs of family members
- ☑ Cooperate with news media personnel

WORDS AND PHRASES YOU MAY BE SEEING FOR THE FIRST TIME

Command post. A place in which the officer in charge of an emergency situation can meet with other emergency service and community resource personnel. May be in a vehicle or a nearby building. Should have communication links with the dispatch center and other services.

Command post kit. A briefcase, trunk, or other container filled with maps, standard operating procedures, directories, community resource lists, inventories, and other items that will help an officer best utilize emergency service forces at the scene of a large-scale incident.

Cul-de-sac. A dead-end street, usually provided with a turnaround at the end.

Ground cover. A tarpaulin that is placed on the ground for an equipment layout.

Parking area. A street or parking area where vehicles not needed in the rescue operation may be safely parked.

Staging area. A street or parking area where ambulances, rescue vehicles, and fire apparatus that are essential to the rescue effort are parked.

Supply point. An area close to the accident site where tools and appliances vital to the rescue effort are stockpiled.

variety of activities designed to support the rescue effort may be required at the scene of a trench accident.

How soon support activities are begun depends on how many rescuers and other emergency service personnel are on the scene. If there is a shortage of manpower, it may be necessary for the officer in charge to delay the start of support operations until hazards are controlled and rescuers have started to make the trench safe. On the other hand, when there are enough emergency service workers on the scene, support activities can be undertaken as soon as the officer completes his assessment.

When a single workman is buried under a relatively small pile of dirt, the rescue effort generally can be accomplished in 1 hour or less. But when one or several workmen are buried under tons of earth, as when a 30-foot long section of spoil pile or a wall slides into a trench, the rescue operation may take many hours.

If it appears that the rescue will be a long-term operation, you should set up and maintain a command post.

ESTABLISHING A COMMAND POST

You can use your rescue unit as a command post; however, if there is a construction office trailer on the job site, it may better serve your need (Figure 5-1). At the very least, it will offer working room that will not be available in the cab or crew compartment of a rescue vehicle and will be removed from the sometimes frenzied activity of the immediate rescue site.

Another advantage of an office trailer is that it will probably have one or more telephones. With your portable radio and the telephones, you will have several communication links that will allow you to talk with other rescuers on the scene, the dispatch center, and community resources.

Still another advantage of maintaining your command post in an office trailer is that you will have the profile and cut sheets on hand at all times. This is important if you have asked the job foreman to accompany you throughout the operation.

Remember
A command post does not have to be directly adjacent to or even in view of the rescue site. Command posts at major fire scenes are often located as far away as several blocks from the involved buildings.

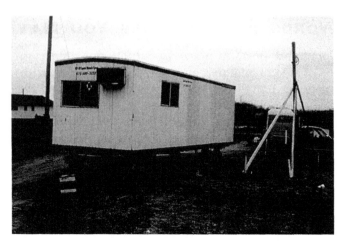

Figure 5-1. An office trailer.

A command post kit (CP kit) is a valuable tool for a long-term operation such as a complex trench rescue effort. A CP kit might include telephone directories, street directories, inventories of equipment, standard operating procedure manuals, pre-plan guides, maps, hazardous material guides, community resource lists, and similar documents. A complete CP kit can be included in a top-loading salesman's case or a large attaché case and carried in a compartment.

Rescue units often carry a flag that identifies the command post. One can be made easily by attaching a brightly colored flag or pennant to a staff that is secured to a magnet. The fluorescent staff and pennant for bicycles that is sold in most auto supply stores makes an excellent command post indicator.

Because there may be many vehicles responding to the scene of a complex trench accident, you need to create a parking area.

CREATING A PARKING AREA

The roads around construction sites are often crowded with construction materials, contractors' trucks, and earth-moving equipment. If there is an influx of emergency vehicles, the roadways to and from the accident site may become completely blocked, delaying vehicles that are carrying equipment vital to the rescue effort.

Many incoming emergency vehicles—especially engines and trucks—only carry personnel to the scene and are not needed at the accident site. Find an area where these vehicles can be safely parked. A cleared area, side streets that are at right angles to the main access road, and cul-de-sacs are good choices.

While you are establishing a parking area, also find a stopping place for rescue vehicles that are essential to the rescue operation.

CREATING A STAGING AREA

Ambulances and rescue vehicles that are used for transportation (and those that must remain in service during the rescue effort) should be directed to a staging area. Find a clear space that connects with the main access road. Assign someone to the task of keeping nonessential vehicles out of the staging area.

If the ground is wet, make sure that neither of the parking areas is so muddy that vehicles become stuck.

CREATING A SUPPLY POINT

If you must rely on other emergency service units or community resource agencies for supplies and equipment, be sure to leave open an area close to the rescue site where supplies and equipment can be organized and distributed. A good rule to follow when deciding where to stockpile equipment is to keep it at least twice the distance from the trench lip as the trench is deep. If the ground at the supply point is muddy, have rescuers lay down ground covers so that small tools will not be lost in the muck.

CONTINUING TRAFFIC CONTROL MEASURES

Access to the rescue site must be denied to all but emergency units throughout the entire operation. Otherwise the many spectators' cars that are often common at an accident scene will prohibit the movement of essential vehicles.

If you assigned rescuers to traffic control tasks during hazard control activities, request that police officers take over. If there are not enough police officers on the scene, delegate traffic control tasks to capable persons such as REACT members or truck drivers.

CONTINUING CROWD CONTROL MEASURES

Once spectators are moved back, they should be kept at a safe distance from the trench. If you previously detailed rescuers to control the movement of bystanders, have those rescuers tie rope barriers at a suitable distance from the rescue site. If you are in an urban area, ask the street and sewer department or the water department to erect barricades to control the crowd.

CONTINUING DEWATERING OPERATIONS

If either a well-point or deep-well system is being used by the contractor to draw off ground water, it must be kept operating during the rescue procedures. Ground water can fill a trench quickly. Ask the job foreman to assign one of the workers to the dewatering system. This will ensure that fuel tanks are kept full, or that electrical services are not disrupted, depending on the type of system being used.

If you had a portable pump installed to remove water from the trench during hazard control activities, make sure that someone refuels the pump from time to time. Have a standby pump available in case the primary one stops and cannot be restarted. Use only electric submersible pumps in the trench. All gasoline- or diesel-fueled pumps must be located outside the trench. Make sure exhaust systems cannot contaminate the trench or blower intakes. Take care that discharge lines from dewatering systems and portable pumps do not flood apparatus–parking areas.

If an accident occurs close to the contractor's quitting time, the rescue effort may continue until after dark. Therefore it may be necessary to provide lighting.

LIGHTING THE SCENE

If darkness falls before rescue operations are finished, you will need lights so that rescuers can work safely and effectively. All lighting needs should be filled a few hours before sunset. Do not wait until the last minute.

Light the immediate rescue site, as well as the command post, the equipment supply point, and the essential vehicle staging area. The parking area for nonessential vehicles should also be illuminated to discourage thieves and vandals. Light and power for the parking, staging, and equipment areas usually can be provided by the parked vehicles. Portable floodlights and extensive cable probably will be unnecessary.

Use at least four 1000-watt floodlights to illuminate the trench and the area around it. Position the lights as high as possible, either on stands or tripods. Place two lights on each side of the trench, close to the ends. In this way they will light the trench, but they will not interfere with the movement of rescuers working at the side of the opening.

Have two or three generators available at the scene of a trench accident so that there is no need for long cables. With more than one generator, there will not be a complete loss of lighting if a generator fails during critical rescue efforts. Nor will there be a loss of power to any vital electrically operated pumps or blowers.

CONTINUING TO MONITOR THE ATMOSPHERE IN THE TRENCH AND PROVIDING FRESH AIR

Methane gas may be present in any trench, and methane is both a flammable gas and an asphyxiant. Be sure that the blower unit installed to ventilate the trench is kept in operation throughout the entire rescue effort.

PROTECTING THE TRENCH DURING INCLEMENT WEATHER

Rain, sleet, and snow can make life miserable for rescuers during a trench rescue operation. Discomfort is not the only consequence of rain, however; rain can seriously affect the integrity of the sheeting and shoring. In inclement weather you should consider erecting a tent-like structure that will keep the elements from the victims, the rescuers, and the devices that are supporting the trench walls. A large salvage cover will serve the purpose.

Lay a 12-foot-long, 2-inch by 12-inch plank across the trench supported by the uprights, so that the plank becomes a ridge pole. Lay the salvage cover over the ridge pole (Figure 5-2). Use this procedure also for setting up a sunscreen.

If water is running into the trench from uphill, have a rescuer build a 6-inch-high dike with dirt from the spoil pile. This will divert water away from the opening. Have the rescuer cover the hem of the tarpaulin that is over the spoil pile as well, to prevent dirt from washing into the trench.

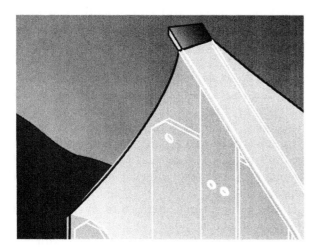

Figure 5-2. A tent covering a trench.

SUPPORTING THE RESCUERS

If the cave-in is extensive and the rescue operation will be prolonged, you will have to rotate digging crews every 10 or 15 minutes. Rescuers tire quickly when they must fill and lift buckets of dirt that weigh 50 pounds or more, especially in a hot, humid environment. Rotating crews will require manpower, so do not hesitate to call for additional personnel even though you do not need additional equipment.

See that rescuers are refreshed during extensive operations. Provide high-protein foods and real fruit juices. See that rescuers have hot drinks and hot soup during cold weather operations, and that they have some sort of shelter for breaks, even if it is nothing more than a salvage cover made into a canopy.

While you are considering the human element of the rescue operation, also consider the need to provide support for the family members of victims.

SUPPORTING FAMILY MEMBERS

It is only natural for family members and friends to rush to the scene when they hear of the accident. A prolonged rescue effort will be a difficult time for these people, especially when hope turns into despair as the operation drags on.

Ask clergymen or personnel from such family service agencies as the Red Cross and the Salvation Army to care for family members and friends during the rescue operation. Although family members may resist, ask the clergymen or service workers to escort them away from the immediate work area. Distraught relatives have a serious effect on rescue workers, who can feel pressured into working in an unsafe way just to conclude the operation. If the rescue looks as if it will be prolonged, you might consider allowing the families to have contact with the victims periodically via portable radio. This would help both parties.

COOPERATING WITH THE NEWS MEDIA

Good public relations are not important to a disaster operation, they are essential! One unfortunate interview with a news reporter can damage a fire department's or rescue squad's image that results from years of good work.

As the rescue officer, you should not take time from the important decision-making process to speak with the news media. Assign a capable officer or squad member to this task. Tell this person to provide the media with an accurate account of the operation, but caution against giving out the names and addresses of injured or missing workers. There is nothing worse than having family members learn the plight of a loved one from the radio or television.

Honor the requests of photographers and television news camera operators if you can, but do so only if they will not get in the way of the rescuers or otherwise pose a threat to the operation, or invade the victim's privacy. Do not allow direct shots that show a victim's face.

Remember

Once started, support operations may have to be continued throughout the entire rescue effort. Be sure that you have sufficient manpower for these important services.

THE PARKWAY INCIDENT—
SUPPORT OPERATIONS

Your squad members have controlled the hazards that you discovered during your assessment of the situation and are now making the trench safe with sheeting and shoring. It does not appear that the operation will be extensive, since one workman is visible and one is buried in a relatively small area.

If the cave-in had been extensive, however, and a number of workmen had been buried, you probably would have elected to initiate a number of support activities.

Indicate on the rescue site plan where you would establish the following equipment and personnel points. Indicate in the spaces provided why you chose those locations.

Command post _____

_____

Parking for nonessential vehicles _____

_____

Staging area for essential vehicles _____

_____

Supply point for tools and equipment _____

_____

It may grow too dark for rescuers to work safely. Indicate on the rescue site plan where you would place generators and floodlights. If you choose to use portable generators, indicate from which units the generators will be taken. _____

_____

Indicate on the plan where you would establish an assembly point for relatives and family service personnel. Why did you choose that location? _____

_____

Indicate on the plan where you would establish an assembly point for news media personnel. Why did you choose that location? _____

_____

Gaining Access

KNOWLEDGE OBJECTIVES

The rescuer should be able to—

- ☑ Define relevant words and phrases
- ☑ Summarize the activities of the "gaining-access" phase of a trench rescue operation
- ☑ List at least three mechanisms of entrapment other than dirt
- ☑ Explain why a backhoe or other machine should not be used to dig for persons who are buried in a trench
- ☑ Describe the procedure for reaching a person through a large-diameter pipe
- ☑ Describe the procedure for reaching a person by hand digging
- ☑ Describe procedures for removing timbers and lengths of pipe in an effort to reach a trapped person
- ☑ Explain the importance of removing dirt from a person's chest as well as his face
- ☑ Describe the procedure for reaching a person who is trapped under a length of pipe
- ☑ Describe the procedure for reaching a person who is trapped under a boulder
- ☑ Describe the procedure for reaching a person who is trapped under a machine
- ☑ List at least four situations in which it may not be possible to make a trench safe with sheeting and shoring
- ☑ Describe the procedure for reaching a trench accident victim by digging to the angle of repose

SKILL OBJECTIVES

The rescuer working individually or as part of a team should be able to—

- ☑ Reach a person through a large-diameter pipe
- ☑ Reach a trench accident victim by hand digging
- ☑ Remove timbers from on top of an accident victim
- ☑ Remove a length of pipe from on top of an accident victim
- ☑ Remove a boulder from on top of an accident victim
- ☑ Remove a machine from on top of an accident victim
- ☑ Reach an accident victim by digging to the angle of repose

WORDS AND PHRASES YOU MAY BE SEEING FOR THE FIRST TIME

Catch basin. A precast or built-in concrete box that is generally used in storm sewer construction.

Choke. To pass the end of a wire rope sling through the eye of the other end and pull it until it fastens securely around the object that is to be lifted.

Choker. Another term for wire rope sling.

Cribbing. Short pieces of lumber used to support and stabilize an object.

Eye of the sling. A loop fashioned into the end of a wire rope.

Mechanism of entrapment. Any object that confines (or traps) an accident victim.

Operating radius (of a crane). The horizontal distance from the centerline of rotation (the center pin of the cab) to a vertical line through the center of gravity of the load.

PVC pipe. A lightweight pipe made of polyvinylchloride.

Shackle. A U-shaped piece of round steel that is provided with a pin or a threaded bolt. Used to join rigging devices.

Once life-threatening hazards have been controlled, the trench has been made safe, and support operations have begun, rescuers can direct their attention to reaching buried victims.

A trench accident victim can become trapped in a number of ways, including:

- By dirt, as when the spoil pile slides in or when a wall collapses
- By sand or stone, as when bedding material is accidentally dumped into the trench, or when a boulder slides into the trench
- By dirt and a section of pipe, as when a section of pipe is dislodged by a pile slide or a wall collapse
- By a length of large-diameter pipe
- By a piece of heavy equipment that topples into the trench
- By improperly installed sheeting and shoring dislodged by the forces of moving earth

Trench accidents can be categorized as involving the movement of earth, or as not involving the movement of earth. Consider the first of these.

ACCIDENTS WITH A CAVE-IN

Gaining access to buried persons may not be an easy task. More than a ton of dirt may have to be moved just to reach a victim whose location in the trench is known. Many tons of earth may have to be removed if the cave-in is extensive and there is no way for rescuers to know where a person is buried.

To gain an idea of the magnitude of the problem, suppose that an accident occurs in a trench that is 4 feet wide by 12 feet deep by 30 feet long. A 4-foot section of one entire trench wall shears away. That is almost 1450 cubic feet of earth weighing over 145,000 pounds! If the location of a buried workman is not known, the entire amount of earth may have to be removed.

> **Remember**
> A backhoe should never be used to free a person who is buried in a trench.

A workman was completely buried when one wall of the trench in which he was working collapsed. The backhoe operator thought he knew exactly where the workman was, so he swung the bucket over the area and took a bite. Undoubtedly, he was thinking that if he could remove a portion of the dirt, it would be easier for the other workmen to

reach the victim with shovels. However, when the bucket bit into the earth, it cut the buried man in half.

In another part of the country at another time, a workman was buried up to his neck in a standing position. The backhoe operator could see the victim in this case, so he thought it would be safe to scoop away dirt from in front of the man so perhaps he could wiggle free. The operator extended his bucket a little too far, unfortunately, and when he went to dig, he tore the man's head off.

When there has been a wall collapse or a spoil-pile slide into a trench that has large-diameter pipe, you should ascertain whether or not there may be a live workman inside the pipe.

REACHING A PERSON THROUGH THE END OF A LARGE-DIAMETER PIPE

An experienced workman may try to dive into the end of a large-diameter pipe during a spoil-pile slide or cave-in. If this occurs, have a rescuer try to make contact with the person from the last manhole or catch basin. If the rescuer is able to hear or see the workman, you may be able to effect the rescue through the pipe. This procedure is not recommended if the pipe is less than 48 inches in diameter. Also, do not attempt a pipe rescue if more of the victim's body is trapped outside the mouth of the pipe unless you are experienced in tunneling.

If you feel that you can complete the rescue through the pipe, remember that you must treat the pipe as you would any confined space and wear a breathing apparatus. Also purge the area with your blower. A supplied-air system is ideal for this sort of operation; there is no weight to contend with, and there is no bulk.

When attempting to rescue a victim trapped in a pipe, wear a safety harness with a retrieval line. Have your backup rescuer remain in the manhole or catch basin. He should be wearing a self-contained breathing apparatus (SCBA) as well if the system is closed and there is a chance that the air may be contaminated. You will also have to take a supplied-air system to the victim.

First, crawl into the pipe. Help the victim into the breathing apparatus and make sure that he is breathing properly. Pass him and dig dirt from around his legs with a small folding shovel. You actually will be tunneling for a short distance without any means of supporting the tunnel roof and walls, so be careful. Spread the dirt that you remove over the floor of the pipe. As soon as the victim's legs and feet are free, pull him into the safety of the pipe.

If you find that the victim is trapped in running

sand, you will have to abandon the attempt and reach him by digging down into the trench. Have someone stay with the person while the digging is accomplished.

If the victim cannot be freed by a rescuer working inside the pipe, or if the victim cannot be seen at the end of the pipe, it will be necessary to dig by hand in an effort to reach him.

REACHING A PERSON BY HAND DIGGING

Hand digging should be accomplished with small shovels such as military-style trenching tools. If a rescuer uses a long-handle shovel or spade in the usual manner, that is, by pushing it into the ground with his foot, he may push the sharp edge into the buried person and inflict a serious wound. Another reason for using a small shovel is that shoring will interfere with the use of one with a long handle.

Do not allow rescuers to throw dirt out of the trench ditch-digger style. When you know where the person is buried—within a relatively small area of earth—instruct rescuers to throw the dirt into the section of the trench that is not affected by the cave-in. When you do not know where the person is, however, do not allow rescuers to dispose of the dirt in this way. They might do nothing but add dirt to that which is already covering the victim.

If you cannot see the bottom of the original trench, all the dirt must be removed. You can find the trench floor by measuring from the engineer's stake, cut sheets, teeth marks in the trench bottom, or stone bedding.

If the dirt must come out, have the rescuers shovel it into 5-gallon plastic buckets, and have rescuers at the edge of the trench lift the buckets to ground level with ropes.

On the ground they can dispose of the dirt on the spoil pile or somewhere else away from the trench. Make sure that the buckets are not lifted directly over the rescuers working in the trench. Remember that buckets full of dirt can weigh more than 50 pounds, and that ropes and bail handles can break.

If the victim is only partially buried, as George is in the Parkway Incident, instruct rescuers to dig carefully around him until he is completely uncovered. To prevent injury, do not allow the rescuers to pull on the victim until all of the dirt has been removed.

REMOVING ANY MECHANISM OF ENTRAPMENT

Once you have a victim partially uncovered, you may find that dirt is not the only mechanism of entrapment. The workman may also be pinned by a length of pipe, a piece of timber, or even a shovel.

Freeing a person from beneath a piece of timber

or a shovel will present no problem; simply cut the object with a saw. Removing a length of pipe may be difficult and time consuming. (We are speaking here of new pipe that was being laid, not pipe that was in the ground before the job.)

Pipes come in lengths from 5 to 20 feet. If it does not seem likely that you can free the person without moving a large quantity of dirt, have rescuers cut the pipe with a power saw that is fitted with the appropriate blade. Be sure that the victim and the rescuers are adequately protected. They should be provided with respiratory protection if it is likely that the cutting operation will produce a great deal of dust. See that cuts are made at a safe distance from the trapped person. Make sure that ventilation of the trench is continued throughout the rescue effort.

UNCOVERING A PERSON'S HEAD AND CHEST

It is natural for rescuers to work feverishly to uncover a person's head, and then slow their efforts once they see that he is alive. You must continue working to uncover his chest. Although the airway can be cleared and oxygen administered when a victim's head is free, he may not be able to breathe properly until the weight of the dirt is removed from his chest.

ACCIDENTS WITHOUT A CAVE-IN

You may at some time respond to a trench accident that has not involved a cave-in. You may find a person under a pipe, under a boulder, or even under a piece of heavy equipment that has toppled into the trench.

WHEN A VICTIM IS TRAPPED UNDER A PIPE

Pipes of a variety of sizes and weights are laid in trenches. Eight inch–diameter PVC pipe is commonly used in underground installations. This is a very strong, lightweight plastic pipe; one workman can easily carry a 20-foot section. If a length of PVC pipe falls onto a man's legs, either he or another workman can lift it. On the other hand, a 20-foot section of 8-inch ductile iron pipe weighs about 650 pounds. If a section of this pipe pins a workman's legs, it will have to be lifted with a backhoe or crane.

Concrete pipes can range in size from 12 inches to 60 inches, and can weigh between 750 and 10,000 pounds. There are several techniques for lifting a concrete pipe that has pinned a workman to the wall or floor of a trench. See the "T" trench scenario in Phase 4, in which the victim is freed with high-pressure air bags.

Most concrete pipes in the 12- to 60-inch range have holes in the center of the side wall, which can facilitate lifting. If the hole is facing straight up, rig the pipe for lifting by first passing the eye of a wire rope sling through the hole. Pass a steel bar through the eye of the sling from the end of the pipe. Catch the other eye of the sling with the lifting hook on a backhoe or crane. Signal the operator to make the lift. If the hole is not facing straight up, do not attempt to lift the pipe in this way. As a strain is taken on the sling, the pipe may roll onto the victim.

Another technique is to pass one eye of a long wire rope sling through the pipe from the end. Join the eyes and catch the lifting hook of the backhoe or crane. Signal the operator to make the lift.

Still another method is to choke the pipe with a wire rope sling. This involves digging under the pipe, however, and that can be a slow and difficult task. It may be the technique that poses the least threat to the victim, however.

> ### Remember
> These techniques are rigging techniques. If you attempt them you should be familiar with rigging practices, and you should have the proper equipment, including an assortment of wire rope and nylon slings, chains, shackles, and come-alongs. Know the capacities of your equipment; moreover, be able to judge the weight of the object that must be lifted or moved.

When a Victim is Trapped Under a Boulder

If a large rock or boulder traps a person, rescuers face a challenge because there is nothing on a boulder to which rigging can be attached.

If you have a wide nylon sling available, use it to lift the boulder. Pass the sling around the stone, making sure that the sling is around the central portion. Choke the sling and attach it to the lifting hook of a crane or backhoe and signal the operator to make the lift.

If you have only wire ropes and chains, place two or three pieces of 2- by 4-inch lumber between the wire rope or chain and the boulder. The pieces of lumber will help prevent the rope or chain from slipping. Choke the sling and catch the eye of the sling with the lifting hook of the machine. Do not try to raise a boulder with a basket lift; it will probably slip.

Instead of trying to lift a heavy and unwieldy boulder, it may be better to try and move it with a jack. Clear enough space under the stone for several pieces of 2- by 12-inch plank; these will serve as a solid base for the jack. Position the jack between the stone and the jack plate and extend it. As the boulder moves, have rescuers install cribbing so that if the jack slips, the stone will not. Move the stone

only far enough for the rescuers to pull the victim free.

When a Victim is Trapped Under a Machine

Be prepared for unusual trench accident situations. You may arrive on the scene to find a loader nose-down in the trench and on top of the operator. If you do, you can be reasonably sure that the accident happened in this way: The loader was being used to dump bedding stone into the trench. The operator allowed his "cats" to extend too far over the edge of the trench. The law of gravity prevailed, and the machine tilted forward. The sudden movement of the machine caused the operator to pitch forward into the trench. The machine followed and pinned him to the dirt floor.

In this type of accident, it does not matter if the trench was made safe with sheeting and shoring or not. As a machine slides into the trench it will collapse the shoring and push the sheeting into the trench.

In situations like this, it is recommended that you neither try to jack the machine away from the victim nor attempt to lift it with a backhoe. Attempting to lift or move a machine with a jack will not be successful unless you are familiar with the location of jacking points. A backhoe will not have the lifting capacity for the job. Now is a good time to put your community resource utilization plan into operation.

Notify your dispatcher that you need a crane at the accident site. Provide him with this information:

- The depth and width of the trench
- The type of soil
- The dimensions of the work area
- The proximity of overhead hazards (wires, trees, etc.)
- The make and model of the machine that must be lifted (if you cannot determine this from a decal or nameplate, ask the job foreman or instruct the dispatcher to call the contractor's office)
- The position that the machine is in (on its side, nose-down, on its top, etc.)

This information is as important to the official of a crane rental company or a construction company as initial information about an accident is to you. On the basis of the information provided, the company official can make a decision as to the size of the crane needed.

Unless you are construction-oriented and well versed in rigging practices, do not ask for a certain-sized crane, such as a 50-ton unit. Just because a crane is rated at 50 tons does not mean that it can life 50 tons in all situations. The ability of a crane to lift depends on many things, including the "operating radius," or the horizontal distance from the centerline of rotation (the center pin of the cab) to a vertical line through the center of gravity of the load. The crane will be able to lift a full 50 tons when the boom is nearly vertical, but as the operator booms out (and the operating radius is increased), the lifting capacity is reduced. Let the expert decide what crane is best suited for the job.

While you are waiting for the crane to arrive, have rescuers sheet and shore the remaining portion of the trench so that when the machine is lifted, they will be able to complete the rescue from a safe area.

When the crane is in place and ready for the lift, clear all of your personnel from the trench. When the machine has been moved to a safe place, have the rescuers finish sheeting and shoring and then prepare the victim for removal.

WHEN A TRENCH CANNOT BE MADE SAFE

There are circumstances under which it is not possible to use sheeting and shoring to make a trench safe for a rescue effort. Such conditions include—

- Slough-in
- When the trench is deeper than 15 feet
- When the soil around the trench is too unstable
- When there has been a massive cave-in that has involved both walls and the entire spoil pile

- When workmen are buried in running sand
- When site conditions are unfavorable, as when obstructions or ground conditions prevent an approach to the accident site with emergency equipment

In any of these situations, it will be necessary to dig to the angle of repose, or, in other words, to slope the ground in such a way that soil will not slide into the rescue area.

Figure 6-1 shows the ground slopes for various types of soil. Be aware that these angles of repose are approximate and that the figures are provided as a guide. In a real situation, it will be necessary to excavate away from the trench boundary to a point where there is no more movement of the soil. For a trench that has been dug 15 feet in sandy soil, the excavation may have to extend to each side for more than 35 feet.

The following procedure is suggested for times when you cannot make a trench safe by any of the methods described earlier.

DIGGING TO THE ANGLE OF REPOSE

Suppose that several workmen are trapped at the bottom of a 30-foot-long trench that has been dug 10 feet deep in sandy soil. Both trench walls have collapsed and the spoil pile has slid in as well. There is nothing but a shallow depression to mark the accident area.

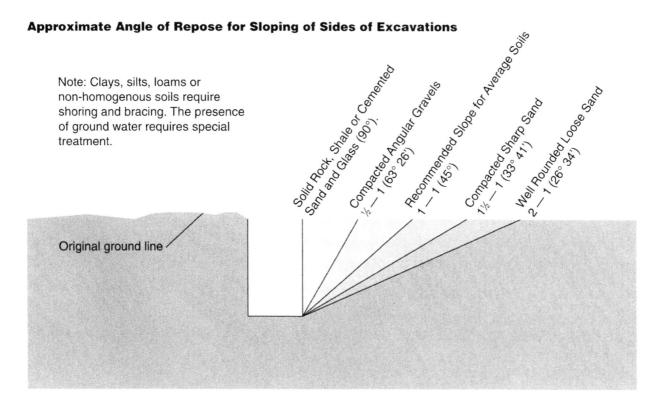

Approximate Angle of Repose for Sloping of Sides of Excavations

Note: Clays, silts, loams or non-homogenous soils require shoring and bracing. The presence of ground water requires special treatment.

Solid Rock, Shale or Cemented Sand and Glass (90°).

Compacted Angular Gravels ½ — 1 (63° 26')

Recommended Slope for Average Soils 1 — 1 (45°)

Compacted Sharp Sand 1½ — 1 (33° 41')

Well Rounded Loose Sand 2 — 1 (26° 34')

Original ground line

Figure 6-1. Angle of repose.

Before you start any digging operations, however, consult with the job engineer about the location of any underground utilities that might be within the rescue area. If the job engineer is not immediately available, try to learn the location of buried utilities through the one-call system.

First, determine the centerline of the trench. Mark the centerline from one end of the caved-in area to the other. Use stakes and a marker that is highly visible, such as yellow polyethylene rope or yellow perimeter tape.

> **Remember**
> The centerline can be determined from the position of manholes and catch basins, the location of the backhoe with relation to manholes, and, most important, from the engineer's hubs.

Determine the width of the trench. Ask the job foreman or the backhoe operator. If neither is available, or if neither knows how wide the trench is, determine what size pipe is being laid. Many utility contractors establish trench width by a rule of thumb, allowing 1 foot of space between the pipe and the trench wall. If a 12-inch pipe is being laid, the trench will probably be 36 inches wide. A trench for 24-inch pipe will probably be 48 inches wide, and so on. When you have determined the width of the trench, define the probable trench boundaries by placing a marker stake on each side of the centerline.

Next, establish the digging lines. Place stakes and marker ropes or tapes 2 feet beyond the trench boundary markers on both sides of the centerline and extend the digging line markers over the entire caved-in area. If you decide that the trench is 4 feet wide, place the digging line markers 4 feet from the centerline, thus marking an area of ground 8 feet wide. The 2-foot buffer zone on each side of the trench boundary will minimize the possibility of the backhoe's bucket touching the victims during the excavation procedure.

Instruct the backhoe operator to pull dirt away from the digging line until the excavation reaches the angle of repose. He should dig as deeply as the trench was dug. If no one is sure of the depth of the trench, consult the engineer's hubs or the cut sheets or profile sheets. When the backhoe operator finishes excavating one side, have him move to the other side and repeat the digging. If you are not sure exactly where the workmen are buried, it is best to excavate the entire length of the caved-in portion.

When the ground is sandy and loose, soil between the digging lines will probably slough into the newly dug area. This will be beneficial; the backhoe will be able to remove soil that would otherwise have to be removed by hand. However, when the soil is compact there may be a solid wall of soil remaining between the digging lines after both sides of the trench are sloped. This, of course, must be removed since the bodies of the victims are underneath.

If the wall is more than 6 feet high, have the backhoe operator gently knock away small portions of the pile at a time, working from the top down. Have him stop near the 6-foot level. Then assign rescuers to climb onto the wall of earth and peel away clumps of dirt with folding shovels.

When all but about 3 feet of the wall remain, warn the rescuers to work carefully; they will be nearing the bodies. Have them continue to dig by hand until the bodies are completely uncovered.

This procedure is time consuming and often difficult. Regardless of how slow the operation seems, don't take short cuts! In a situation like the one described, the chance of survival for the buried victims is very slim. You must not jeopardize the lives of rescuers for a body-recovery operation.

THE PARKWAY INCIDENT—
GAINING ACCESS

Reaching George is no problem; he is only partially buried. Reaching Henry will pose no serious problem since he is known to be buried in a relatively small area of the trench. But suppose you reach Henry and you find that he is trapped by something other than dirt. With the supplies and equipment that you would normally have available at the time of a real trench accident, how would you reach Henry if he were trapped:

Under a pipe? _____

_____

_____

Under a boulder? _____

_____

_____

Under a piece of heavy equipment? _____

_____

_____

At this point we are going to end our joint participation in the Parkway Incident because the information contained in the rest of the book does not lend itself well to the workbook approach.

If you have conscientiously completed the work sections at the end of the first six phases, you should have a good idea of your unit's capabilities for a trench rescue operation. Your time has been well spent!

Emergency Care

KNOWLEDGE OBJECTIVES

The rescuer should be able to—

- ☑ Define relevant words and phrases
- ☑ Summarize activities of the emergency-care phase of a trench rescue operation
- ☑ Describe the steps of in-trench emergency care procedure

SKILL OBJECTIVES

The rescuer working individually or as part of a team should be able to—

- ☑ Carry out in-trench emergency care measures

WORDS AND PHRASES YOU MAY BE SEEING FOR THE FIRST TIME

Cardiac arrest. A sudden cessation of heart action followed by the loss of arterial blood pressure.

Cardiopulmonary resuscitation. The combination of chest compressions and ventilations provided by rescuers in an effort to restore spontaneous breathing and heart action in a person who has suffered cardiac arrest.

Carotid pulse. The rhythmic expansion of the large arteries on both sides of the neck; easily felt with the fingertips.

Cerebrospinal fluid. The clear, watery fluid that helps protect the brain and spinal cord.

Cervical collar. A semi-rigid adjustable collar that partially stabilizes the neck after an injury.

Closed wound. An injury in which the skin is not broken.

Contusion. A bruise.

Crepitation. The crackling sound that is produced when broken bone ends rub together.

Dilated pupils. Widened pupils of the eyes (as opposed to pupils that are narrowed, or constricted).

Evisceration. Disembowelment; protrusion of the organs through an opening in the abdomen.

Extrication collar. A cervical collar with high sides, providing additional protection for the cervical spine.

Jaw-lift method. A technique for opening the airway by displacing the tongue. The rescuer hooks the jaw of the nonbreathing person between his thumb and forefinger and gently lifts.

Jaw-thrust method. Another technique for opening the airway of a nonbreathing person. A forward displacement of the lower jaw by the rescuer causes the tongue to move away from the air passage.

Lackluster pupils. Pupils that are dull, lacking the radiance usually associated with the eye.

Neck lift–head tilt maneuver. Still another technique for opening the airway. The rescuer places one hand under the person's neck and lifts while he presses on the person's forehead with his other hand.

Occlusive material. A nonporous, nonabsorbent material (such as plastic wrap) that is used to seal an open wound and protect it from air.

Open abdominal wound. An injury in which the abdominal wall has been penetrated.

Open wound. An injury in which the skin is broken and underlying tissues are exposed.

Spontaneous breathing. Involuntary, instinctive breathing; breathing that occurs without outside influence.

Sucking chest wound. An opening in the chest wall and underlying lung through which air moves in and out with each respiration.

CARRYING OUT EMERGENCY CARE PROCEDURES

It is important to understand that emergency care in a trench collapse situation is relative to many factors not encountered in non-trench emergencies. The size of the trench may be too small to allow normal emergency care procedures. The victim may be still partially covered and emergency care restricted to his accessible body areas. In any case, emergency care procedures carried out in a trench should be limited to those that preserve life and limit disability.

CLEARING AND MAINTAINING THE AIRWAY WITH CERVICAL SPINE CONTROL

Regardless of the mechanism of injury, it is critical that a victim's airway be cleared of debris and maintained. Rescuers following clearing procedures must remain constantly aware of the possibility of cervical spine injury. Such injury is often caused by the force of a trench collapse. Cervical spine control is best accomplished by a second rescuer supporting the victim's head in a neutral position. If this is impossible, the application of a rigid extrication collar will assist in stabilizing the cervical spine. Remember that a rigid cervical collar alone will not accomplish definitive cervical spine control; it will only assist in stabilization.

It is likely that you will find the victim's mouth full of dirt. He may have been calling for help when the accident occurred, or he may have opened his mouth in an effort to breathe after being covered. The victim's airway may be compromised by bleeding or loose teeth caused by trauma to the head and face. Airway obstruction may consist of vomitus as a result of extreme pressure on the abdominal cavity during the cave-in. The most common type of airway obstruction, although, is the tongue.

The airway of the victim should be opened with the modified jaw-thrust maneuver. Suction should be readily available for obstructions of blood and vomitus. The finger-sweep maneuver should be used for obstructions caused by dirt, teeth, etc. If the victim is unconscious and there is adequate space, consider intubating the trachea to gain definite airway control and assist ventilation.

EXAMINING FOR BREATHING AND PROVIDING VENTILATORY ASSISTANCE

Listening and feeling for air exchange at the mouth and nose may be the best method to determine the presence of respirations. The chest and abdomen may be covered so that they are not accessible for respiratory evaluation. The lungs of an apneic victim may be ventilated without moving the victim. Resuscitation may be best accomplished by the bag-valve-mask unit. A demand-valve ventilator should be used with great care because of the likelihood of chest injuries. Excessive positive-pressure ventilation will accelerate complications such as tension pneumothorax.

If the victim is found to be breathing, supplemental oxygen should be provided with a non-rebreather mask. Remember that if the victim's chest is covered with dirt, or the victim is trapped against a pipe, thoracic expansion will be severely compromised. The use of supplemental oxygen to compensate for reduced tidal volumes may be lifesaving.

EXAMINING FOR CARDIAC FUNCTION AND PROVIDING CIRCULATORY ASSISTANCE

You must be realistic about cardiopulmonary resuscitation (CPR) in a trench collapse situation. Often there will not be enough room in the trench to provide this care. Although you can provide ventilatory support to a victim in an upright position, CPR must be performed with the victim in a supine position. Furthermore, prolonging the time of extrication/access may render such an intervention impractical.

Cardiac status should be assessed at the carotid artery. If space and the position of the victim permit, you may perform CPR as usual.

CONTROLLING SEVERE BLEEDING

Open and closed wounds may be inflicted during the trench collapse. Severe external bleeding may be inhibited by circumferential pressure applied to the body by the collapsing material, or by compression of extremities under a pipe or other heavy object.

External bleeding control can be accomplished by direct pressure on a wound, digital pressure on a pressure point, or by use of a tourniquet. In traditional emergency care, the use of a tourniquet is always limited to bleeding that cannot be controlled by any other method. When faced with a trench rescue situation, a tourniquet may have to be used if the bleeding part cannot be reached because of the position of the victim in the trench. The tourniquet should be a blood-pressure cuff of the appropriate size.

As the victim is dug out of the trench, the rescuer should look for areas of severe bleeding and be ready to provide bleeding control immediately. If a body extremity is pinned beneath a heavy object, such as a pipe, a blood-pressure cuff should be placed, but not inflated, nearest the injury to provide immediate bleeding control upon release of the extremity.

The rescuer must be aware of the possibility of internal bleeding from closed wounds. Look for the signs of shock and be ready to intervene at the earliest possible time with oxygen therapy, volume replacement, and pneumatic anti-shock garment (PASG).

Time should not be wasted trying to bandage all open wounds. Instead, quickly apply direct pressure to a wound with bulky dressings. The dressing may be held in place with a pneumatic splint, which will provide stabilization of the dressing as well as excellent bleeding control.

EXAMINING FOR HEAD INJURY

During a cave-in a victim's skull may be fractured, resulting in injury to the brain. Examine the victim for wounds, bruising, or deformity of the head, as well as unequally dilated pupils and the presence of cerebrospinal fluid in the ears or nose. It is equally important to determine the level of consciousness of the victim.

Care of the victim should include airway clearing with cervical spine protection, bleeding control, and administering high-flow 100% oxygen. In closed head injuries the lungs of the victim should also be hyperventilated to help reduce brain swelling.

EXAMINING FOR INJURIES TO THE CHEST AND ABDOMEN

Chest and abdominal injuries are common in trench collapse situations because of the extreme pressures placed upon these areas by falling dirt and rock.

The chest and abdomen may be penetrated by a number of objects, including tools, pieces of wood, and pipe. If an object is impaled in the victim's flesh, it should be stabilized in place with bulky dressings and tape or cravat bandages.

A sucking chest wound must be sealed with an occlusive-type dressing. Household plastic wrap makes an efficient seal if it is folded several times. The plastic wrap should be applied over the wound and taped in place leaving one corner open to act as a flapper valve. This will allow excess air to escape from the chest and reduce the possibility of tension pneumothorax.

Difficulty in breathing, deformity, failure of the chest wall to expand normally during breathing, tracheal deviation, jugular vein distention, and the coughing up of bright red blood are common indicators of closed chest injury. The rescuer must be alert

to these signs and provide airway control and ventilatory assistance with oxygen.

EXAMINING FOR EXTREMITY FRACTURES

Extremity fractures should be stabilized, as conditions permit, before the victim is removed from the trench. If traditional splints cannot be used, fractured bones of the upper extremity may be fastened to the victim's chest and fractured bones of the lower extremities may be immobilized by tying the legs together.

PROTECTING THE SPINE

Application of a vest-type spinal immobilization device, which is the easiest kind to apply in the confined areas of a trench, will provide adequate stabilization. When you extricate the victim, do not lift him by the vest unless the device is specifically made for lifting.

TREATING HYPOTHERMIA

The victim of a trench collapse may be subject to hypothermia. The temperature of the air and ground, the presence of water, and the length of entrapment time will affect the degree of hypothermia. The rescuer should be aware of these conditions and provide care for the victim. Hypothermia should be considered a potential problem year-round, since the ground temperature remains fairly constant, and in most cases the victim cannot move his extremities or body to generate body heat.

Place hot packs under the victim's armpits. Cover the victim to reduce heat loss, especially wrapping the cover under the victim if possible. If they are available, provide the victim with heated oxygen and warmed intravenous fluids, to warm the core of the body. Heating the trench may be accomplished with the type of heaters used by the telecommunications industry for heating cable vaults. These heaters are propane powered, provide an excellent heat source, and have been proven to be the best heaters available. We have added one to your equipment list in Figure 1-30. Keep in mind that there is no such thing as complete combustion, so you may notice trace amounts of propane on your atmospheric monitor. As long as the LEL and O_2 levels remain stable, keep right on truckin'.

Your community resource list should provide telephone numbers of the local power company or telephone company, both of which operate trucks with this type of heater. In a pinch you can use hot packs and hair dryers. If you choose to use anything electric, make sure you employ a ground fault interrupter (GFI).

Treating Crush Injuries and Crush Syndrome

The impact of collapsing earth is tremendous. If a victim survives this impact, you need to make sure that the extrication effort does not aggravate his injury.

In recent years, study of victims trapped in collapsed buildings after earthquakes has identified issues relating to the injuries caused by the crushing forces of trench collapse and the effect of long-term compression of the body. Also identified as an issue is the sudden release of confined parts of victims' bodies.

A number of things happen when the body is crushed. First and most obvious is the damage to the tissue and bone as a result of the impact. This usually is not visible when you look at the patient, even if you could see the affected area. In fact, it is typical in trench accident situations, including fatalities, for there to be no visible sign of injury on the body.

The second effect is crush injury, which increases as the time that the area is without oxygenated blood increases. Crush injury causes death of the tissue in the affected area. The time required for this to become a problem can be as short as 1 hour if the compression is severe. But even with less severe pressure, you can be assured of crush injury within 4 to 6 hours.

The third problem is crush syndrome, which occurs when the victim is freed and the injured tissue releases fatal toxins into his blood stream. As long as the toxins are confined in the injured area, the victim can survive. But when the victim is released and the toxins move to the vital organs, the victim's heart typically stops. This phenomenon has given rise to the sometimes-heard term "grateful dead syndrome;" a live victim can appear grateful for rescuers' efforts but, unfortunately, die as soon as he is freed from entrapment.

What can you do as a rescuer to avoid crush syndrome? First, and most important, recognize that it is a potentially life-threatening condition. Next, make sure that your local medical community is knowledgeable about the problem and trained in the proper field treatment. In most cases, paramedics trained in crush syndrome can provide the care required to save a crushed victim's life. The key is that the care must be started before release.

The treatment provided will probably include a rapid-flow intravenous line, various medications, monitoring of the EKG abnormalities, and O_2—preferably humidified. Any course of treatment must be determined by health care professionals trained in the treatment of crush injuries.

Disentanglement

KNOWLEDGE OBJECTIVES

The rescuer should be able to—

☑ Define relevant words and phrases
☑ Summarize activities of the disentanglement phase of a trench rescue operation
☑ Explain the reason for not attempting to pull a person free from the trench floor with a rope
☑ Describe the procedure for freeing a person by hand digging
☑ Describe the procedure for supplemental sheeting and shoring when the level of the trench floor is lowered by digging
☑ Describe procedures for removing water that enters a trench during the digging operations
☑ Describe the procedure for adjusting sheeting and shoring installed against frozen ground

SKILL OBJECTIVES

The rescuer working individually or as part of a team should be able to—

☑ Free a person from the floor of a trench by hand digging
☑ Supplement sheeting and shoring as digging lowers the level of the trench floor
☑ Remove water that enters the trench during the digging operations
☑ Adjust sheeting and shoring when frozen ground thaws

WORDS AND PHRASES YOU MAY BE SEEING FOR THE FIRST TIME

Bedding stone. Small rocks spread over the floor of a trench as a foundation for sewer pipes and other utility lines.

Cathead. A shore running between walers with a 6-inch-longer plank nailed to the top.

Diaphragm pump. A positive displacement pump that has a diaphragm instead of a piston; an excellent device for moving water in which foreign matter is suspended.

Frost line. The depth to which frost penetrates the soil.

Manifold. A pipe fitting with several inlets and/or outlets.

Spot dewatering. The technique of drawing water from localized portions of the ground around a trench.

Sump. A small pit dug at the lowest point in a trench floor; it serves to keep the screened end of a suction hose below the water level.

Supplemental sheeting and shoring. Additional sheeting and shoring installed as the level of the trench floor is lowered during digging operations.

Surcharge. Additional weight in the trench area.

Water table. The upper limit of the portion of ground that is wholly saturated with water from underground source. May be near the surface or many feet below.

In many vehicle accidents the victim does not need to be disentangled. If a person is not trapped, simply opening the vehicle may free him. Such is often the case in trench rescue operations. If a workman is buried horizontally, digging to him will free him from the dirt that is trapping him.

FREEING A VICTIM COMPLETELY

Gaining access will not always result in freeing a trench accident victim, however. A separate disentanglement step may be necessary. Consider the case in which a workman is buried in a standing position.

During the "gaining-access" phase the victim is uncovered to a point below his waist so that emergency care procedures can be initiated. With the patient care operations underway, only the task of freeing the person's legs remains.

An untrained rescuer might immediately decide to slip a rope under the person's arms and have rescuers at ground level pull him free. Because of the weight of the dirt around his legs, and the suction that is often common to wet ground, such an effort may result in the separation of joints in the victim's hips and legs. If this happens with a manual operation, think of the damage that might be inflicted if the untrained rescuer attached the rope that is under the person's arms to the lifting hook of a backhoe bucket. Ghastly as it may sound, a person could actually be pulled apart in this manner. Obviously, the correct procedure is to dig to get the victim free.

DIGGING BY HAND

Disentanglement should be accomplished in the same manner as gaining access—by rescuers using small folding shovels.

Dig a foot or so away from the person's legs so that there is no chance of cutting them with the shovel. Toss the dirt onto the trench floor some distance from you, or, better yet, have it removed from the trench altogether by bucket. When you are within a few inches of the person's legs, move the dirt with your hands. Simply pull it into the excavation that you have made with the shovel. Continue to pull dirt away from his legs and feet until they are completely uncovered.

By all means, resist any thoughts of digging for a person by using machinery.

DIGGING BY MACHINE

Consider this scenario: A utility contractor was laying pipe in an unshored trench dug 7 feet in sand. One of his workmen was trapped in a standing position when both side walls of the trench caved in. The workman was not injured and, since he was buried only to his waist, he was having no trouble breathing. As a matter of fact, he was talking and joking about his predicament while other workmen were trying to free him.

The foreman felt that the work was not going fast enough, however, and he decided that the rescue could be accomplished more quickly with the backhoe. He felt that if the operator were to dig well away from the trapped workman, the other workmen could push the sand into the excavation and thus speed the operation.

In his anxiety to free the trapped workman, the foreman forgot about the water main that bisected the trench. The backhoe bucket ruptured the main, and everyone stood by helplessly while the water flowed up to and then over the trapped victim's head, drowning him.

> **Remember**
> Do not control hazards, make a trench safe, carefully reach and care for a trapped person, and then place the whole rescue operation in danger by attempting to do with a machine what should be done by hand.

Two pieces of equipment have been added to our inventory in recent years: the air knife (Figure 8-1) and the vacuum truck. The air knife was mentioned in Phase 4, and was used to cut out the sides of the trench walls to accept outside walers.

The air knife was developed for locating and clearing underground utilities. It will only penetrate porous materials such as dirt; it will not harm solids such as fiberoptics or, for that matter, anything underground. Because of this, it is an excellent tool for breaking dirt away from buried persons. It can be used as a probe and will not harm a victim. It operates at 125 psi with 150 cfm. The venturi mechanism boosts the velocity of the air to mach 2, or 1700 mph, while the discharge pressure is reduced to about 90 psi. The velocity of the machine tears apart the earth.

Always be sure to wear eye and hand protection when working with an air knife. It is a power tool; treat it as such.

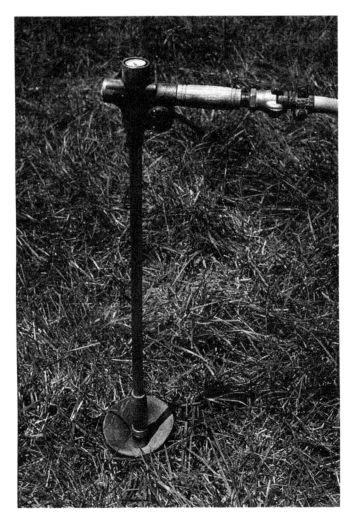

Figure 8-1. An "air knife."

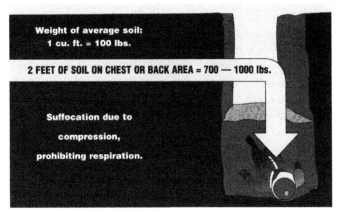

Figure 8-2. Weight of soil.

The vacuum truck used for catch basin and manhole cleaning is ideal for sucking out the loose material created by employing the air knife or by hand digging. It eliminates having to remove dirt from the trench. This machine is quite powerful, so be careful when placing your hands near the end of the suction tube. It will handle small rocks as well as dirt. Do not try to pick up large solids because the tube can become clogged. The truck should be backed up to the trench only after the trench is sheeted and shored. The truck becomes surcharge loading, which could directly affect the "safing" of the trench.

SUPPLEMENTAL SHEETING AND SHORING

The disentanglement phase of a trench rescue operation may include more than just the digging efforts. There may be a need to supplement the sheeting and shoring so that the digging and victim removal activities can be carried out in safety.

Suppose that you have properly sheeted and shored a trench that is 10 feet deep after a slide of the spoil pile. The original trench was 15 feet deep, however, so you know that the victim is buried somewhere in the 5 feet of dirt below the new floor of the trench. The victim could be just below the surface of the floor, he could be lying on the original floor, or he could be buried in a sitting position some 3 feet below the surface. He could be anywhere.

For the purpose of illustrating the need for supplemental sheeting and shoring, imagine that the victim is lying prone with about 3 feet of dirt covering him (Figure 8-2).

As rescuers remove the dirt in their effort to reach him, they will be exposing the trench wall below the sheeting and shoring. By the time they can free the victim, they will have exposed from 2 to 3 feet of trench wall. They also will have created the potential for disaster!

When more than 2 feet of trench wall remains unsupported, there is the distinct possibility of a slough-in, and a slough-in at the bottom of a trench will initiate a chain reaction. The slough-in creates a void below the bottom edge of the sheeting. If the soil is less than compact, it will flow from behind the sheeting into the open space below. A new and larger void will be created behind the sheeting. With no support for the sheeting, the panels and shores will become loose and the whole structure will collapse on the rescuers. Therefore, it is necessary to supplement the original sheeting and shoring whenever more than 2 feet of trench wall is exposed during the digging operation.

To go back to the beginning, when you arrive on the scene and see that there is neither a medical emergency nor the pinning of a victim, but rather a burial, you know that you will be digging to free the victim or recover a body.

Once the trench has been sheeted and shored, you should immediately plan on installing walers. Walers serve two purposes: they provide strength, and they open the area making it easier to work.

On every job, make it a standard operating procedure to install short (2- by 12- by 12-inch) scabs on the uprights immediately above the shores, being careful not to lock in the shores (Figure 8-3).

This procedure ensures that when the wale is placed in position, there will be enough room behind it to place 2-inch by 12-inch by 12-foot planks vertically (Figures 8-4 and 8-5).

When the walers are positioned, install a "cathead" as a spreader. The cathead should be of the same-dimensioned lumber as the walers. An exception could be a pneumatic jack used in place of a 6-by 6-inch timber. Eight- by 8-inch or 10- by 10-inch walers need the same size cathead (Figure 8-6).

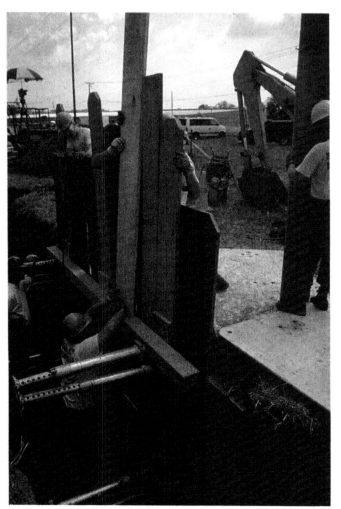

Figure 8-4. Placing supplemental sheeting.

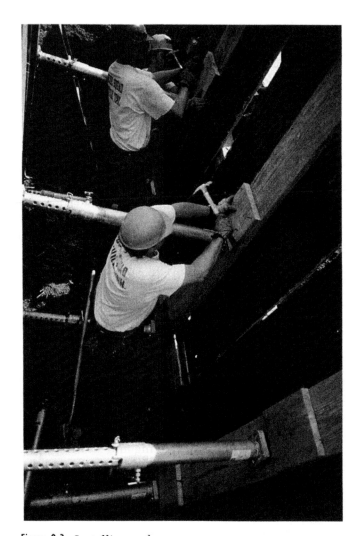

Figure 8-3. Installing scabs.

When building the cathead, spread the walers with a hydraulic jack, ram, or spreader, or use a screw jack with a short piece of pipe (Figure 8-7). Take an exact measurement and cut the appropriate-sized timber. Now lay a piece of 2-inch by the corresponding-sized timber, 6 inches longer than the shore on top of the shore. Nail it on with three nails, leaving 3 inches sticking out on each end (Figure 8-8).

Drop the cathead between the walers and nail one end to hold it in place. Release the pressure on the jacking device and nail the other end (Figure 8-9).

Do not exceed 8 feet between catheads. Remember that all wale sizes are relative to the depth and width of the trench (Figure 8-10).

Now we are ready to install the 2-inch by 12-inch by 12-foot supplemental sheeting. Drop the planks in from the top (Figures 8-11 and 8-12). Three panels will accept eight planks per side (Fig-

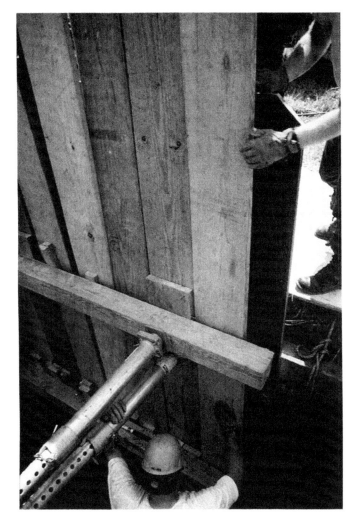

Figure 8-5. Placing supplemental sheeting for a cathead.

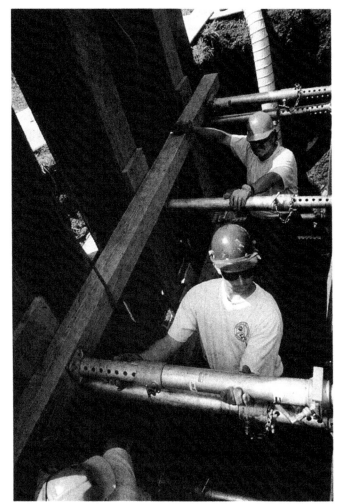

Figure 8-6. Using pneumatic shoring.

ure 8-13). Lock them in with wedges (Figure 8-14). You are now ready to dig (Figure 8-15).

Keep the digging square, that is, from sheeting to sheeting and the length of the "safed" area. Never dig a "V" hoping to detect where the body is. You will not be able to work comfortably in a V-shaped hole.

Once you have dug 2 feet, square off the hole and drop the planks one at a time. Do this by loosening the wedges on one plank, placing a square-nosed shovel with its back toward the plank and close to the wall. As the plank is dropped, push the shovel handle and jam the plank against the wall. Relock it with the wedges. This is a very important step, because the plank will tend to bow into the trench.

Place another set of walers. The catheads should be the same length if you are digging squarely. Repeat this procedure as you work down the trench. The intermediate set of walers can be removed so that you end up with walers every 4 feet.

If for some reason the vertical planking method

cannot be employed, have your men use the following procedure.

As soon as they remove 2 feet of dirt, have them stop and slide two 2-inch by 12-inch by 4-foot

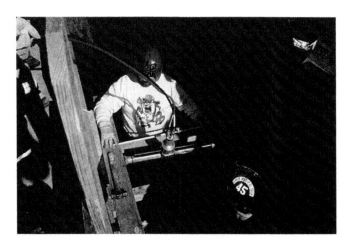

Figure 8-7. Spreading walers for the cathead.

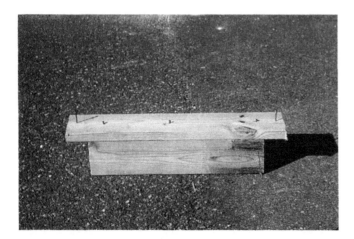

Figure 8-8. Timber cathead.

planks under the uprights of the original sheeting. Thus the solid sheeting will be continued straight down. Do this for every panel on each side of the trench.

Install the proper-sized shore against the upright that is holding the newly installed sheeting in place. Figure 8-16 shows a trench wall against which 2 feet of supplemental sheeting and shoring has been installed.

Install sheeting in this way every time an additional 2 feet of trench wall is exposed. When you must install sheeting below the original uprights, provide supplemental uprights as well as sheeting.

Have the topside crew cut pairs of 2-inch by 12-inch by 2-foot planks. Place them vertically against the 2-inch by 12-inch by 4-foot planks that you have placed horizontally as sheeting. This will ensure that the uprights are continued straight down. Install shores against these new uprights. Figure 8-17 shows a trench wall that has 4 feet of supplemental sheeting and shoring installed.

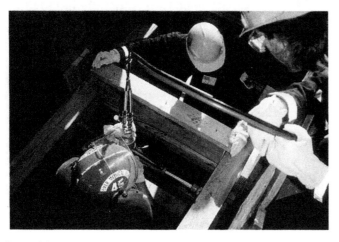

Figure 8-9. Release the pressure on the jacking device.

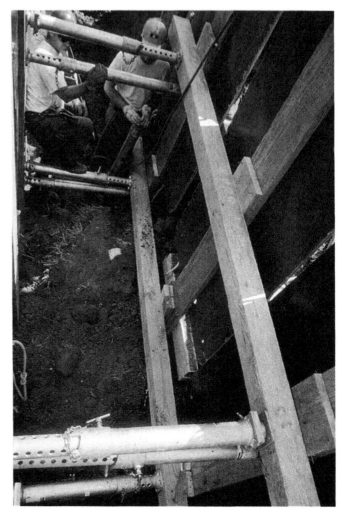

Figure 8-10. Catheads must be 8 feet apart.

> **Remember**
> Never underestimate the need for supplemental sheeting and shoring just because the trench walls "look" safe. Do not make a trench safe only to risk having the entire structure collapse because of the failure of a relatively small section of trench wall during the digging operation.

DEWATERING THE TRENCH DURING DIGGING OPERATIONS

Be prepared for the problem of water interfering with digging and victim removal operations. Water may seep through the lower portions of the trench walls or may actually bubble up through the trench floor. Moreover, you may experience difficulty with water even though the trench walls were relatively dry when you installed the sheeting and shoring.

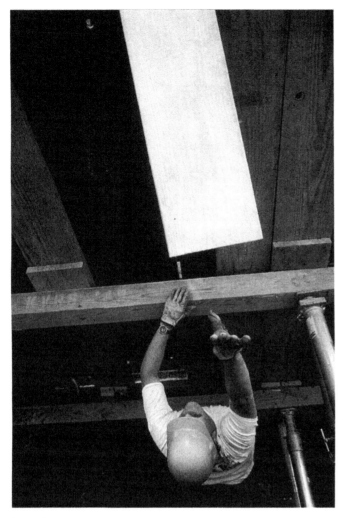

Figure 8-11. Drop in the supplemental sheeting.

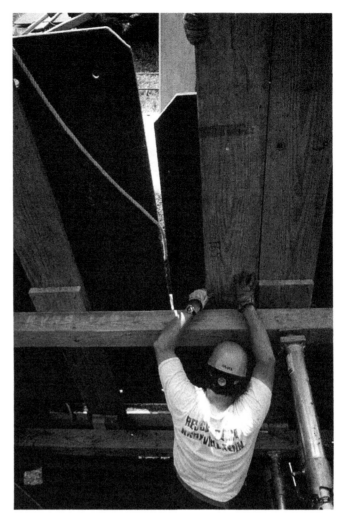

Figure 8-12. Drop in the supplemental sheeting.

Water can come from a number of sources. The water table that is just below the floor of a trench may be reached during the digging operations. Water may be diverted to the trench walls or the ground below the trench floor when water-bearing ground is dis-turbed. Water can also seep into the trench when well-point and deep-well systems fail to keep up with the flow. Whatever the source, water can turn the floor of a trench into a sea of mud that can slow down victim recovery and make the operation dangerous.

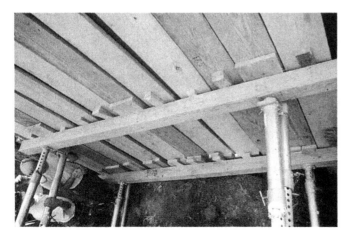

Figure 8-13. There should be eight planks per side.

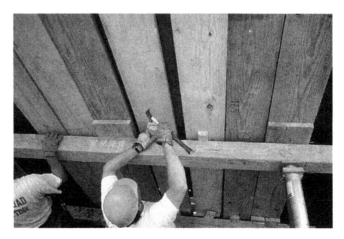

Figure 8-14. Secure the planks with wedges.

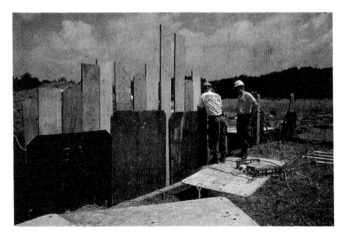

Figure 8-15. Beginning digging.

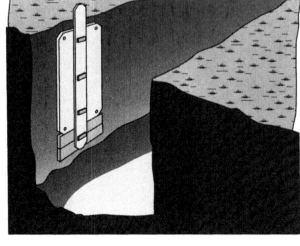

Figure 8-16. Two feet of supplemental sheeting and shoring.

There are two basic ways water can be removed from the floor of a trench. It can be pumped from the trench through a suction hose that rests on the floor, or it can be removed from below the level of the trench floor.

PUMPING FROM THE TRENCH FLOOR

Above-ground-level pumping is easily accomplished. Simply drop a suction hose over the edge of the trench and operate the pump. However, there will always be several inches of water to contend with, depending on the efficiency of the pump and how close the suction strainer is to the floor of the trench. If you must remove water in this way, you can be sure that you will be continually working in mud.

SPOT DEWATERING

Illustrated in Figure 8-18 is a unique device that many contractors use for "spot" dewatering operations—for removing water from small areas of extremely wet sandy soil. The device has a manifold that is connected to the suction side of a diaphragm pump. Four suction lines can be connected to the manifold that is shown. Dewatering is accomplished through 20-foot lengths of flexible suction hose that are fitted with 5-foot lengths of pipe terminating in a spear-shaped well point.

In a rescue operation, the well point (or well points) are pushed into the ground around the victim, and the water is sucked from the soil.

It is suggested that if you live in an area where the ground is sandy and wet and water is likely to be a problem during a trench rescue operation, you

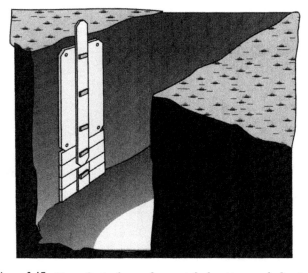

Figure 8-17. Four feet of supplemental sheeting and shoring.

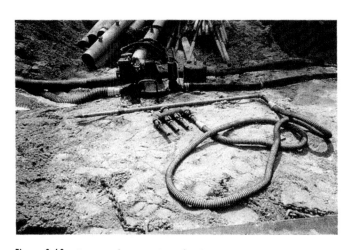

Figure 8-18. A spot dewatering device.

find out which contractors have spot dewatering devices.

MAKING A SUMP

Even if you do not have access to a spot dewatering device, you need not be troubled with any more than a shallow covering of water on the floor of the trench during a rescue effort. Simply build a sump.

Dig a hole approximately 2 feet deep; make it several inches wider than the strainer on the suction hose of your portable pump. Place a few inches of bedding stone in the bottom of the hole. Remember that there will almost always be bedding stone on the site of a pipe-laying job. Lower the suction strainer into the hole. While another rescuer holds the suction hose in the center of the hole, shovel bedding stone between the wall and the hose. The stone will serve as a filter, and the pump will be able to function exactly like a basement sump pump. The pump will not draw water from the soil, but it will minimize the problem of surface water (Figure 8-19). Have the sump dug and suction hose placed regardless of the weather. Then if there is a sudden storm, as on a summer day, you will not be caught short.

ADJUSTING THE SHORING IF THE GROUND IS FROZEN

If you live in a part of the country where the temperature drops below freezing, be aware of a problem that is associated with frozen ground.

When you respond to a trench accident during the cold months, you may note that the ground appears stable. If the trench has been freshly dug, the stable appearance may extend just to the frost line. If the trench had been dug the day before, the stable appearance may extend deep into the trench. In either case, any impression that the soil is compact and the ground is stable may result solely from the fact that the ground is frozen. Freezing "tightens" soil particles and causes them to appear

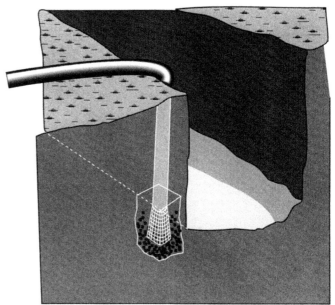

Figure 8-19. A sump hole.

compact. The problem—and the danger—becomes evident after the sheeting and shoring are installed.

When sheeting is placed against a frozen trench wall, the shoring can be installed and tightened to the point at which it appears absolutely rigid. However, when sunshine strikes the sheeting, the panels absorb heat. This heat is transmitted through the relatively thin panels rather quickly, and in turn the heat warms the ground behind the sheeting. As the ground warms, the frozen soil particles soften, and a layer of soft earth forms behind each 32-square-foot panel. Because there is no longer a firm foundation, the panels "give" slightly, and the shores become loose, making the entire sheeting and shoring structure subject to collapse.

You can minimize the problem of frost-caused collapse by having rescuers examine the entire shoring system every 30 minutes to make sure that the shores are tight. When they find that shores have loosened, they can restore the integrity of the system by tightening them.

Removal and Transfer

KNOWLEDGE OBJECTIVES

The rescuer should be able to—

- ☑ Define relevant words and phrases
- ☑ Summarize activities of the removal and transfer phase of a trench rescue operation
- ☑ Describe the procedure for completing in-trench emergency care measures
- ☑ List at least three appliances that can be used for removing an injured person from a trench
- ☑ Describe procedures for securing a person to the various patient-carrying devices
- ☑ Describe the procedure for hoisting a stretcher by means of a hand line and ladder
- ☑ Describe the procedure for hoisting a stretcher with a crane or backhoe
- ☑ Describe the procedure for hoisting a stretcher with an aerial apparatus
- ☑ Describe the procedure for moving a stretcher uphill
- ☑ Describe the procedure for moving a stretcher over rough terrain

SKILL OBJECTIVES

The rescuer working individually or as part of a team should be able to—

- ☑ Complete in-trench emergency care procedures
- ☑ Secure a person to a patient-carrying device
- ☑ Hoist a stretcher by means of a hand line and ladder
- ☑ Hoist a stretcher with a crane or backhoe
- ☑ Hoist a stretcher with an aerial apparatus
- ☑ Move a stretcher uphill
- ☑ Move a stretcher over rough terrain

WORDS AND PHRASES YOU MAY BE SEEING FOR THE FIRST TIME

Backboard. A rigid, full-body immobilization device generally 6 feet long by 18 to 24 inches wide and made of wood; often called a long spine board.

Basket stretcher. A basket-like, formed wire or plastic patient-carrying device designed to afford maximum protection for a person who must be moved over rough terrain.

Hauling line. A length of rope used to hoist or lower an object.

Packaged patient. An injured person who, with wounds dressed and bandaged and fractures immobilized, has been secured to a patient-carrying device.

Reeves Sleeve®. A stretcher-like device that can be used for wrapping a victim or as an immobilization device.

Signalman. A person who gives or relays commands to a heavy equipment operator.

Snatch block. A wood- or steel-shell single pulley block that can be opened on one side to accept a rope or cable.

Tag lines. Handheld lengths of rope—usually $\frac{1}{2}$ inch in diameter—used to steady or move an object that is being hoisted or lowered.

There are two distinct parts to the removal and transfer phase of a rescue operation. During the removal stage, the injured person is secured to a patient-carrying device, or "packaged," and removed from the trench. During the transfer part of the operation, the victim is moved from the edge of the trench to a waiting ambulance.

Both procedures can be somewhat complex. Removing the stretcher-borne person may be difficult because of the depth of the trench and the positioning of the shoring devices. Transfer may be difficult because of the terrain. In some instances, transferring the stretcher will involve no more than the rescuers carrying it over level ground to a nearby ambulance. At times, however, it may be necessary for a number of rescuers to move the stretcher a considerable distance over mounds of earth, piles of construction debris, or other obstacles.

COMPLETING THE EMERGENCY CARE PROCEDURES

When a half-buried person has been completely uncovered, you can examine him for injuries to the lower extremities. If you find injuries, care for them quickly. Again, do not allow the floor of the trench to become an emergency room.

PACKAGING THE PERSON FOR REMOVAL

Any number of patient transfer devices can be used. A Reeves Sleeve® (Figure 9-1), a basket stretcher, or a full backboard is preferred, however. Removal of a person from the floor of a trench will often have to be accomplished with the stretcher maintained in a vertical position because of the shoring devices. All of the patient transfer devices mentioned here are suitable for a vertical lift.

The Reeves Sleeve® is the most desirable device because it provides quick and easy packaging, can be used as a body bag in the cases of body recovery, and can be made rigid by the insertion of a spine board (for those times a "C" spine injury is suspected). It can be hoisted both vertically or horizontally and can be carried readily over rough terrain (Figure 9-2).

> **Remember**
> Under no circumstances should you remove shoring devices so that the stretcher can be lifted in a horizontal position.

REMOVING THE PERSON FROM THE TRENCH

If the trench walls have been dug back to the angle of repose, removing the person will involve little more than four rescuers carrying the stretcher up the slope from the trench floor to the ground level.

If the trench has been made safe with sheeting and shoring, however, the stretcher will have to be lifted to ground level in some fashion. You should never attempt to pass the stretcher or backboard to ground level by hand, nor should you have rescuers raise the stretcher by rope. In either case, if the

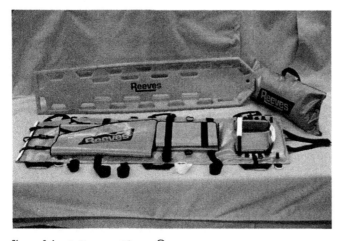

Figure 9-1. A Reeves Sleeve®.

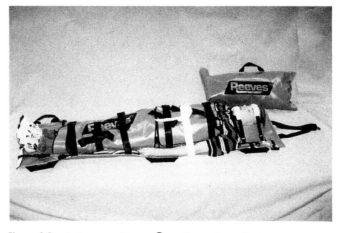

Figure 9-2. A Reeves Sleeve® with packaged victim.

stretcher slips, it can displace shoring, upsetting the integrity of the shoring in places.

HOISTING WITH A HAND LINE AND LADDER

Move the stretcher to a point close to the base of the ladder that is used for entering and leaving the trench. Have rescuers at ground level pass down the end of a hauling line at least $\frac{1}{2}$ inch in diameter. Secure the end of the line to the head end of the stretcher or backboard. Have other rescuers at ground level haul the stretcher or board up. Guide it so that it continually rests on the ladder beams. If the trench is deep, follow the stretcher up the ladder. This will enable you to make sure that the stretcher does not slide from the beams.

USING A CRANE, BACKHOE, OR AERIAL APPARATUS

If there is a crane already set up on the job site, use it to expedite the removal of the stretcher or backboard from the trench. In most cases, cranes and backhoes are not manlifts. You cannot use them for lifting or transferring a person. Use the machines for an anchor point only. Do the rest of the work with your own hauling devices.

Have the crane or backhoe operator swing to the side of the trench so that you can rig a hauling device such as the System 99®, a Haul Safe®, or a block and tackle to the lifting hook. The aerial apparatus should be rigged with the appropriate nylon sling in basket fashion with carabiners to attach the hauling system.

Rig the patient transfer device to the hauling system with an appropriate bridle. Tie two tag lines on the bottom of the device if you are going to make a vertical lift, or on the sides if you are going with a horizontal lift.

Drop the tag lines in the trench to the rescue crew. Swing the machine to the center of the trench and have the crew pull the stretcher down. Have the operator dog-off the machine.

Now you can see the big advantage of installing walers. You will have plenty of room to make a horizontal lift. It is so much easier to package a victim horizontally than vertically. At any rate, you do what you have to do. Let's get on with it!

After packaging, have the top crew start the lift while the trench crew guides the stretcher up through the shoring. When the stretcher is above ground level, instruct the tag line operators to pull it to a safe place as you let off on the hauling system.

TRANSFERRING THE PERSON TO AN AMBULANCE

Once the stretcher is at ground level it can be moved to an ambulance. Two situations may require special movement techniques: when the stretcher must be moved up a hill, or when the stretcher must be moved over mounds of earth or piles of debris.

MOVING A STRETCHER UPHILL

The steeper a hill is, the more difficult it is for rescuers to climb while carrying a stretcher. Here are some suggestions for making the task easier.

One simple method is to extend two ropes down the hill to help rescuers keep their balance when the terrain is rough or the ground is slippery as well as sloped. The ropes should be tied to a firmly fixed object at the top of the hill, about 6 feet apart and 4 feet above the ground. It is important that these suggestions for distance be followed. If the ropes are too close to the ground, rescuers will have to stoop as they pull themselves to the top of the hill.

The other ends of the ropes can be tied to objects at the bottom of the hill, such as trees or vehicles, or two rescuers can be assigned to hold the ropes in place at the proper height. The rescuers carrying the stretcher can then pull themselves up the hill by means of the ropes. If a rescuer loses his footing, another can hold onto the rope while he regains his balance.

Another method is to secure a rope to the head-end of the stretcher and pull it up while rescuers walk beside and support it. The pull can be accomplished with manpower. It may be better to rig the pulling line so that the persons doing the hauling do not have to stand in line with the rope at the top of the hill, however.

Secure a snatch block to a tree, a utility pole, a guardrail, or a vehicle so that the block is about 4 feet above the ground. The block will change the direction of the rope and those persons assigned to haul it can be situated along the crest of the hill where their efforts can be seen and coordinated.

Supervise the pulling operation closely. Have the rescuers hauling the line pull steadily and smoothly in a hand-over-hand fashion. Have them match their pulling speed against the speed of the rescuers ascending the hill.

MOVING A STRETCHER OVER ROUGH TERRAIN

Rather than have four or six rescuers carry the stretcher over rough ground or piles of debris, it may be better to have the stretcher pass from person to person. Simply form two lines of stretcher-bearers. Have them pass the stretcher from hand to hand while they remain in position. When the stretcher passes pairs of individuals, they can leave the rear and go to the head of the line. By leapfrogging in this manner, ten or twelve rescuers can move a stretcher over rough ground or debris for a considerable distance.

The removal and transfer phase of the rescue operation ends when the injured person is placed in the ambulance and the emergency is over!

Termination

PREPARING TO LEAVE THE SCENE
Removing Tools and Equipment from the Trench
Removing Sheeting and Shoring

PREPARING THE UNIT FOR SERVICE

CLEANING AND SERVICING EQUIPMENT
Sheeting
Uprights
Timber Shores
Screw Jacks
Pneumatic Shores
Dewatering Pumps
Power Tools
Rigging
Hydraulic Jacks
Hardware and Hand Tools

COMPLETING THE REQUIRED REPORTS

CRITIQUING THE OPERATION

THE LAST WORD

KNOWLEDGE OBJECTIVES

The rescuer should be able to—

- ☑ Define relevant words and phrases
- ☑ Summarize activities of the termination phase of a trench rescue operation
- ☑ Describe the procedure for removing tools and equipment from the trench
- ☑ Describe procedures for removing sheeting and shoring from the trench
- ☑ Describe procedures for cleaning and servicing equipment used during the rescue effort

SKILL OBJECTIVES

The rescuer working individually or as part of a team should be able to—

- ☑ Remove tools and equipment from the trench
- ☑ Remove sheeting and shoring from the trench
- ☑ Clean and service equipment used during the rescue effort

WORDS AND PHRASES YOU MAY BE SEEING FOR THE FIRST TIME

Boxed end of the shore. The end of a timber shore that is held in place against the sheeting with scabs.

Burr. A rough protrusion from the face of a metal part.

Wedged end of the shore. The end of a timber shore opposite the boxed end. It is between this end and the uprights that wedges are driven to make the structure rigid.

The emergency is over! Victims have been uncovered, removed, and transferred to waiting ambulances. The work of rescue personnel is far from over, however. During this last phase of the operation, rescuers must recover equipment, return to quarters and carry out whatever steps are required to make the unit ready for the next call.

PREPARING TO LEAVE THE SCENE

Keep one point foremost in your mind when you are terminating activities at the scene of a trench accident: the trench will pose a continuing threat to rescuers until they are away from it.

If you follow an orderly sequence of operations from the time that you arrive on the scene until the victims are removed from the trench, follow an equally orderly plan as you prepare to leave the scene.

REMOVING TOOLS AND EQUIPMENT FROM THE TRENCH

Have rescuers in the trench hand up tools and equipment, or have rescuers at ground level haul up tools in the dirt buckets.

Instead of putting the tools on the rig as soon as they are recovered, however, have the rescuers lay them out on the ground cover at the supply point. This will allow you and the driver to see that everything has been removed from the trench.

REMOVING SHEETING AND SHORING

Great care must be exercised during this phase of termination activities. Removing the materials that were installed to make a trench safe should not be a "snatch and grab" operation that is undertaken just so that everyone can go home. It must be a methodical procedure during which the sheeting and shoring materials are removed in precisely the reverse order in which they were installed. In other

Remember

Have rescuers work in the protected area at all times, just as they did when they were making the trench safe. Do not allow them to take short cuts. There is a real danger that the trench walls will collapse when the support that has been provided by the sheeting and shoring is no longer present.

words, the last shore placed is the first shore to be removed.

As rescuers prepare to pull the last supporting shores free with ropes, have everyone who is not essential to the operation move away from the trench. Instruct the rescuers who are removing the last shores to step back quickly if there is any movement of the trench wall or the ground under them.

If a tool or shore drops into the now-unprotected trench as the last piece of shoring is removed, either leave it or reinstall a section of sheeting and shoring so that it can be retrieved safely. No tool or shore is so valuable that a rescuer is justified in jumping into an unprotected trench after it. It would be tragic to lose a rescuer in such a way, especially after the squad has completed a textbook operation.

If a trench rescue operation has lasted long into the night, it might be better to have the squad return in the morning to remove the sheeting and shoring. They will be able to work in the daylight, and they will have had a chance to rest. If you choose to do this, be sure to secure the rescue site to keep people away from the open trench. In the morning, make certain that the sheets and shores are tight before allowing rescuers to descend into the trench.

Let us consider some specific techniques for removing sheeting and shoring.

A WALL SHEAR, SPOIL-PILE SLIDE, OR SLOUGH-IN

You will recall that in situations of wall shear, spoil-pile slide, or slough-in, the walls of the trench on both sides remain vertical or almost vertical.

REMOVING SHEETING AND TIMBER SHORES

Follow these step-by-step procedures:

Step 1. Remove the shores from the last pair of panels installed.

> **Remember**
> The last shore in is the first shore out. The rescuer removing these shores can work from the still-protected portion of the trench.

Step 2. Remove the panel from the side opposite the spoil pile first.

Step 3. Keep the immediate work area clear by carrying the panels to the supply area.

Step 4. Have a rescuer on the spoil-pile side of the trench push the second panel across the trench. If the trench is wide, have him secure a rope and pass the rope across the trench so that other rescuers can pull the panel across the trench.

Step 5. Remove the second panel, and continue to remove sheeting and shoring in this way until only one pair of panels remains.

Step 6. Remove the top scabs from the boxed end of each shore.

Step 7. Have crew members hold the panels in place so that they will not slip sideways.

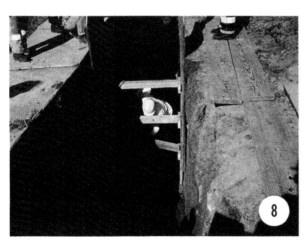

Step 8. Remove the bottom shore and move up the ladder.

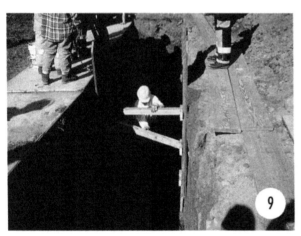

Step 9. Remove the center shore.
◄

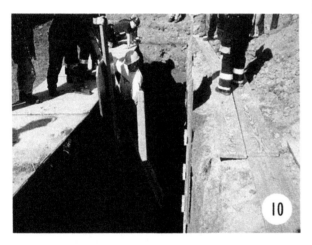

Step 10. Remove the top shore by hand as you come out of the trench.
◄

Step 11. Have crew members remove the last pair of panels from the trench.

REMOVING SHEETING AND SCREW JACKS

Remember to reverse the order of installation.

Step 1. Remove the top shore from the last pair of panels installed.

Step 2. Remove the bottom shore.

Step 3. Remove the center shore. Move to a safe area and have rescuers remove the pair of panels. Continue to remove sheeting and shoring in this way until only one pair of shored panels remains.

Step 4. Remove the bottom shore.

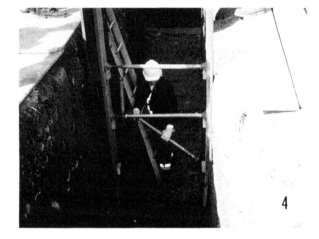

Step 5. Move up the ladder. Remove the center shore.
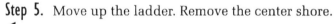

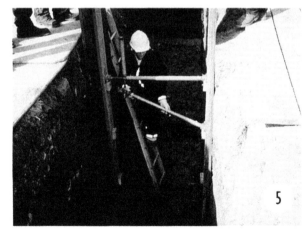

Step 6. Loosen the top shore. Remove it as you climb from the trench.
◄

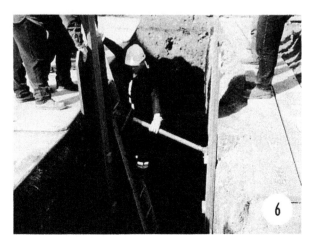

Step 7. Have rescuers remove the last pair of panels from the trench.

REMOVING SHEETING AND PNEUMATIC SHORING

Step 1. While rescuers topside hold the panels in place, remove the top, bottom, and center shores in that order. Step into the safe area of the trench and hand the shores to a rescuer at the trench lip.

Step 2. Have rescuers remove the first pair of panels.

Step 3. Remove the next pair of panels in the same manner. Continue to remove shores and panels until only one pair of panels remains.

Step 4. Remove the bottom shore from the last pair of panels, then the top shore. Pressurize the center shore, loosen the T-handle, attach the hook of the lifting and lowering rope to the T-handle, and remove the pin. It is important that the rescuer operating the air valve maintain a constant pressure on the shore until the rescuer working with the shores is out of the trench. ◀

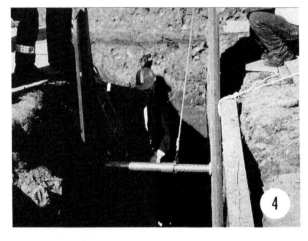

> **Note**
> In some instances, when the pin is nearly vertical, you can attach the hook directly to the top of the pin, thus leaving the pin in place until you are out of the trench.

Step 5. Climb from the trench.
◀

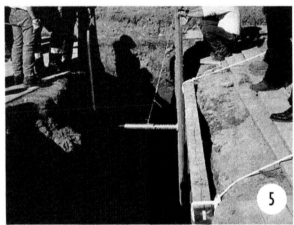

Step 6. Have rescuers hold the panels in place. Instruct the rescuer operating the valve to release the pressure in the shore. Pull the shore from the trench and then remove the panels. ◀

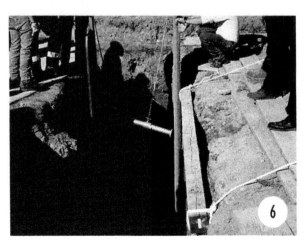

"T," "L" AND "X" TRENCHES, AND SHALLOW WELLS

The sheeting and shoring removal procedures just described were listed in step-by-step fashion for a reason: there were certain important points to be made, such as the way that pressures in pneumatic shores are released. Since special steps required for removal operations have been made clear, we will simplify the instructions for removing sheeting and shoring when they are used in conjunction with a wale or wales: remove the panels and shores in exactly the reverse order in which they were installed!

PREPARING THE UNIT FOR SERVICE

A number of maintenance operations are in order once the unit has returned to quarters.

CLEANING AND SERVICING EQUIPMENT

If your unit has its own sheeting and shoring devices, have squad members care for them in this manner:

SHEETING

It is important to check for damage that has made panels unserviceable.

- Wash each panel thoroughly. Dirt can hide cracks just as wood putty can hide cracks in furniture.
- Examine each panel for fractures. If you see a fracture, remove the panel from service.
- Sand away any splinters.
- Repaint scraped areas.

UPRIGHTS

As is the case for sheeting, cracks in uprights cause them to be dangerous.

- Wash each upright thoroughly.
- Examine each upright for fractures; discard any that are unserviceable.
- Examine each upright for sections in which many nails have been driven. Many nail holes in a small area weaken the wood.
- Re-treat scraped areas.

TIMBER SHORES

- Replace any timber shores that are less than 8 feet long.
- Save pieces of timber that are longer than 36 inches.

- Examine for checks and cracks and timbers that can be salvaged.

SCREW JACKS

- Examine the swivel ends and make sure that they turn freely.
- Examine the screw portion of each jack for burrs that will interfere with their adjustment. Remove any burrs with a file.
- Clean each shore with a wire brush.
- Do not oil screw jacks. Oil attracts dirt, and dirt interferes with the operation of the jack.

PNEUMATIC SHORES

- Disassemble each unit by removing the piston from the barrel.
- Swab the interior of each barrel with soapy water.
- Wash exterior surfaces with soapy water.
- Allow the parts to dry and reassemble the shores.
- Check the air supply for proper operation.
- Be sure that each air coupling is clean.
- Check for operation.

DEWATERING PUMPS

- Clean and service according to the operating manual.
- Check the oil, and change the oil if necessary.
- Check the suction hose for cuts, and clean the suction strainer.
- Refill the gasoline safety can.

POWER TOOLS

- Clean and service each tool.
- If the chain saw was used, sharpen the blade.
- Refill the safety can with the proper mixture of gas and oil.

RIGGING

- Check each wire rope sling and choker for cuts, kinks, burrs, and frayed ends.
- Check synthetic-fiber ropes for cuts, abrasions, fiber pulls, and melting.
- Check the screw pins of shackles for burrs.
- See that block sheaves turn freely.
- Check the hooks of hoisting equipment for spreading.
- Inspect chains for stretching.
- Clean the chains with a wire brush and spray them with a rust preventative.

HYDRAULIC JACKS

- Clean exterior surfaces with soapy water.
- Check the fluid level, and refill if necessary with the correct hydraulic fluid.
- Check for proper operation.

HARDWARE AND HAND TOOLS

- Replenish the nail supply so that there are at least 10 pounds of double-head nails on hand. Discard used nails.
- Replace 2- by 4- by 6-inch wood scabs. Save used scabs for training classes.
- Replace split wedges.
- Clean ground cloths.
- Clean and examine ladders.
- Clean and service hand tools.

COMPLETING THE REQUIRED REPORTS

Fill out response reports according to your unit's SOP guide. Be accurate, and make sure that all parts of the forms are completed. Your reports may be examined thoroughly if there is a formal investigation of the accident or if lawsuits are filed at some later date.

CRITIQUING THE OPERATION

As soon as practical after-maintenance chores are complete and the unit is ready for service, assemble all of the personnel who were involved and review the rescue operation. Give everyone the opportunity to speak, and record their observations and suggestions. Because of such critiques, subsequent rescue operations are conducted more efficiently.

THE LAST WORD

The thought of a trench rescue is intimidating to a great many fire and rescue personnel. It shouldn't be! Appreciate the dangers of an open trench. Prepare your unit for the task either by equipping it or by knowing the availability of community resources. Train your people. Then, when the call comes in, follow the prescribed steps while using common sense and safe practices. Do all that and a trench rescue will be no more difficult than a rescue from a structure or a vehicle. The intent of this book is to guide you step by step in procedures quite foreign to most rescuers. The book is for ready reference on how to accomplish hands-on training; it is not a substitute for hands-on training. Only by doing these tasks over and over will you become proficient, confident, and safe in the overall. Let's go home.

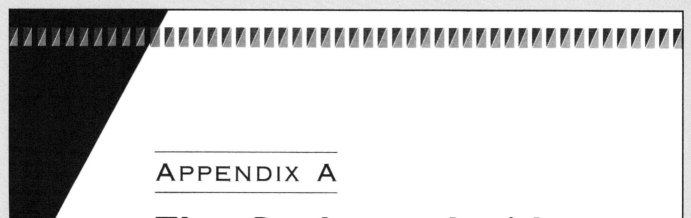

APPENDIX A

The Parkway Incident

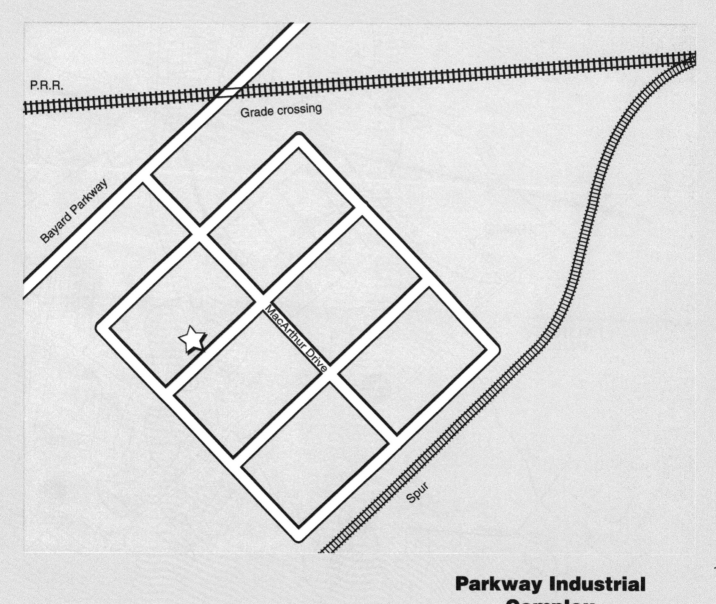

Parkway Industrial Complex

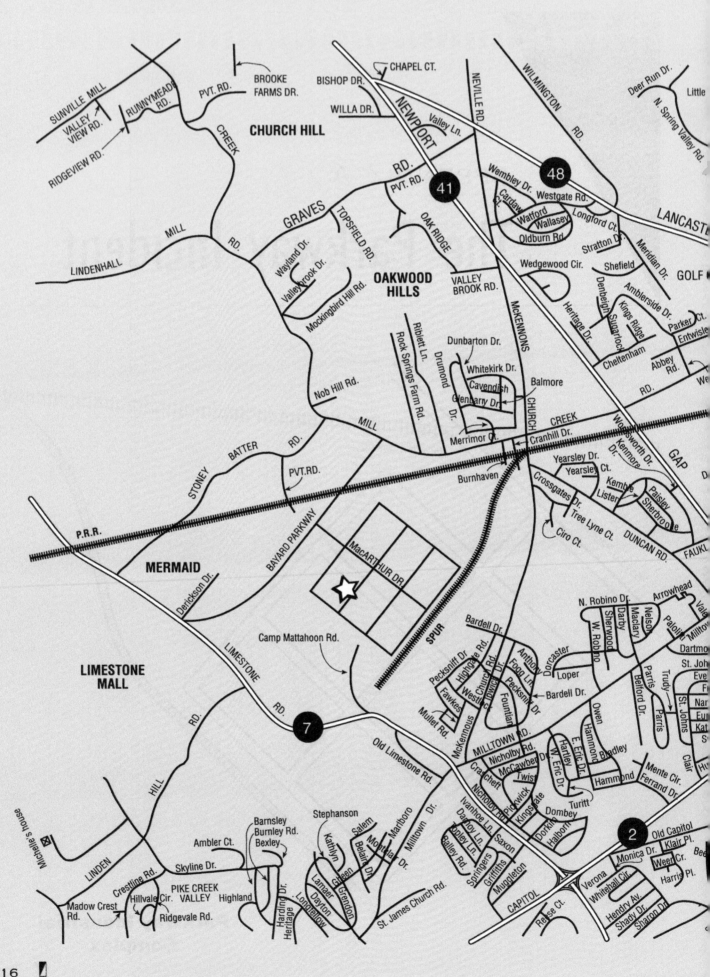

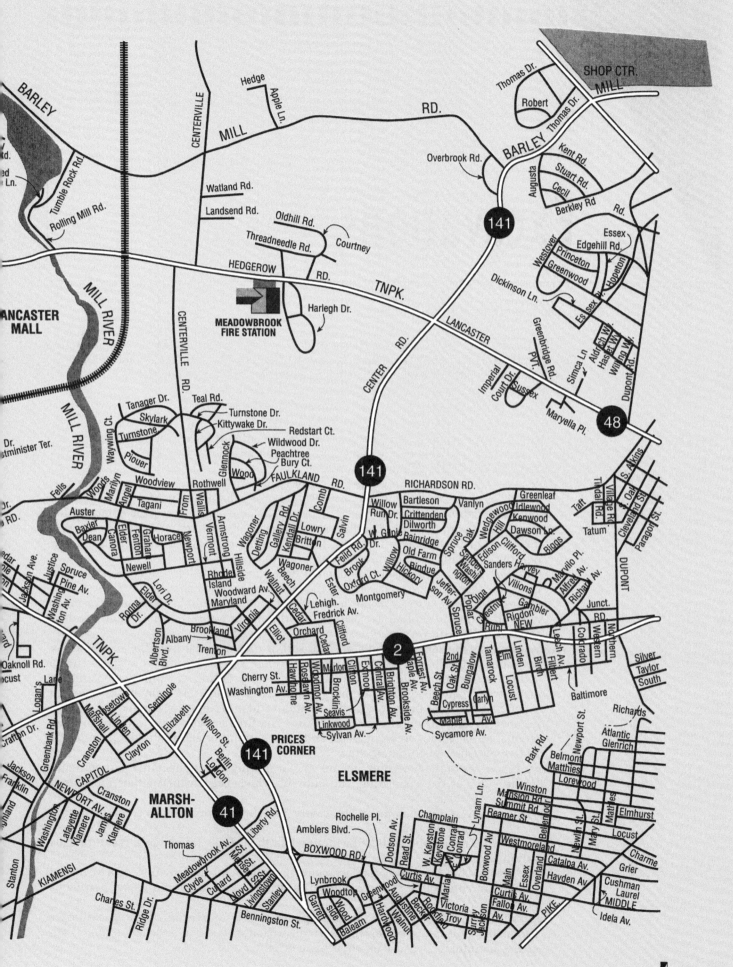

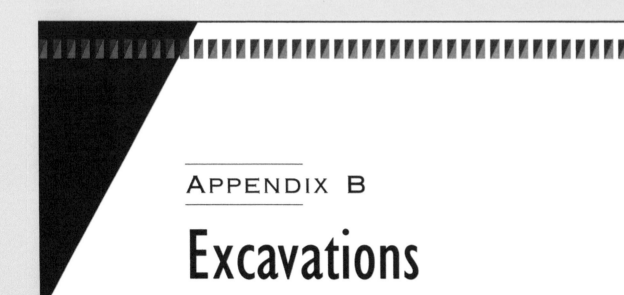

Appendix B

Excavations

(From Subpart P—OSHA 29 CFR Ch. XVII)

Authority: Sec. 107, Contract Worker Hours and Safety Standards Act (Construction Safety Act) (40 U.S.C. 333); Secs. 4, 6, 8, Occupational Safety and Health Act of 1970 (29 U.S.C. 653, 655, 657); Secretary of Labor's Order No. 12-71 (36 FR 8754), 8-76 (41 FR 25059), or 9-83 (48 FR 35736), as applicable, and 29 CFR part 1911.
SOURCE: 54 FR 45959, Oct. 31, 1989, unless otherwise noted.

§1926.650 Scope, application, and definitions applicable to this subpart.

a. *Scope and application.* This subpart applies to all open excavations made in the earth's surface. Excavations are defined to include trenches.

b. *Definitions applicable to this subpart.*

Accepted engineering practices means those requirements which are compatible with standards of practice required by a registered professional engineer.

Aluminum Hydraulic Shoring means a pre-engineered shoring system comprised of aluminum hydraulic cylinders (crossbraces) used in conjunction with vertical rails (uprights) or horizontal rails (walers). Such system is designed, specifically to support the sidewalls of an excavation and prevent cave-ins.

Bell-bottom pier hole means a type of shaft or footing excavation, the bottom of which is made larger than the cross section above to form a belled shape.

Benching (Benching system) means a method of protecting employees from cave-ins by excavating the sides of an excavation to form one or a series of horizontal levels or steps, usually with vertical or near-vertical surfaces between levels.

Cave-in means the separation of a mass of soil or rock material from the side of an excavation, or the loss of soil from under a trench shield or support system, and its sudden movement into the excavation, either by falling or sliding, in sufficient quantity so that it could entrap, bury, or otherwise injure and immobilize a person.

Competent person means one who is capable of identifying existing and predictable hazards in the surroundings, or working conditions which are unsanitary, hazardous, or dangerous to employees, and who has authorization to take prompt corrective measures to eliminate them.

Cross braces mean the horizontal members of a shoring system installed perpendicular to the sides of the excavation, the ends of which bear against either uprights or wales.

Excavation means any man-made cut, cavity, trench, or depression in an earth surface, formed by earth removal.

Faces or sides means the vertical or inclined earth surfaces formed as a result of excavation work.

Failure means the breakage, displacement, or permanent deformation of a structural member or connection so as to reduce its structural integrity and its supportive capabilities.

Hazardous atmosphere means an atmosphere which by reason of being explosive, flammable, poisonous, corrosive, oxidizing, irritating, oxygen deficient, toxic, or otherwise harmful, may cause death, illness, or injury.

Kickout means the accidental release or failure of a cross brace.

Protective system means a method of protecting employees from cave-ins, from material that could fall or roll from an excavation face or into an excavation, or from the collapse of adjacent structures. Protective systems include support systems, sloping and benching systems, shield systems, and other systems that provide the necessary protection.

Ramp means an inclined walking or working surface that is used to gain access to one point from another, and is constructed from earth or from structural materials such as steel or wood.

Registered Professional Engineer means a person who is registered as a professional engineer in the state where the work is to be performed. However, a professional engineer, registered in any state is deemed to be a "registered professional engineer" within the meaning of this standard when approving designs for "manufactured protective systems" or "tabulated data" to be used in interstate commerce.

Sheeting means the members of a shoring system that retain the earth in position and in turn are supported by other members of the shoring system.

Shield (Shield system) means a structure that is able to withstand the forces imposed on it by a cave-in and thereby protect employees within the structure. Shields can be permanent structures or can be designed to be portable and moved along as work progresses. Additionally, shields can be either premanufactured or job-built in accordance with §1926.652 (c)(3) or (c)(4). Shields used in trenches are usually referred to as "trench boxes" or "trench shields."

Shoring (Shoring system) means a structure such as a metal hydraulic, mechanical or timber shoring system that supports the sides of an excacation and which is designed to prevent cave-ins.

Sides. See "Faces."

Sloping (Sloping system) means a method of protecting employees from cave-ins by excavating to form sides of an excavation that are inclined away from the excavation so as to prevent cave-ins. The angle of incline required to prevent a cave-in varies with differences in such factors as the soil type, environmental conditions of exposure, and application of surcharge loads.

Stable rock means natural solid mineral material that can be excavated with vertical sides and will remain intact while exposed. Unstable rock is considered to be stable when the rock material on the side or sides of the excavation is secured against caving-in or movement by rock bolts or by another protective system that has been designed by a registered professional engineer.

Structural ramp means a ramp built of steel or wood, usually used for vehicle access. Ramps made of soil or rock are not considered structural ramps.

Support system means a structure such as underpinning, bracing, or shoring, which provides support to an adjacent structure, underground installation, or the sides of an excavation.

Tabulated data means tables and charts approved by a registered professional engineer and used to design and construct a protective system.

Trench (Trench excavation) means a narrow excavation (in relation to its length) made below the surface of the ground. In general, the depth is greater than the width, but the width of a trench (measured at the bottom) is not greater than 15 feet (4.6 m). If forms or other structures are installed or constructed in an excavation so as to reduce the dimension measured from the forms or structure to the side of the excavation to 15 feet (4.6 m) or less (measured at the bottom of the excavation), the excavation is also considered to be a trench.

Trench box. See "Shield."

Trench shield. See "Shield."

Uprights means the vertical members of a trench shoring system placed in contact with the earth and usually positioned so that the individual members do not contact each other. Uprights placed so that individual members are closely spaced, in contact with or interconnected to each other, are often called "sheeting."

Wales means horizontal members of a shoring system placed parallel to the excavation face whose sides bear against the vertical members of the shoring system or earth.

§1926.651 General requirements.

a. *Surface encumbrances.* All surface encumbrances that are located so as to create a hazard to employees shall be removed or supported, as necessary, to safeguard employees.

b. *Underground installations.*

1. The estimated location of utility installations, such as sewer, telephone, fuel, electric, water lines, or any other underground installations that reasonably may be expected to be encountered during excavation work, shall be determined prior to opening an excavation.

2. Utility companies or owners shall be contacted within established or customary local response times, advised of the proposed work, and asked to establish the location of the utility underground installations prior to the start of actual excavation. When utility companies or owners cannot respond to a request to locate underground utility installations within 24 hours (unless a longer period is required by state or local law), or cannot establish the exact location of these installations, the employer may proceed, provided the employer does so with caution, and provided detection equipment or other acceptable means to locate utility installations are used.

3. When excavation operations approach the estimated location of underground installations, the exact location of the installations shall be determined by safe and acceptable means.

4. While the excavation is open, underground installations shall be protected, supported or removed as necessary to safeguard employees.

c. *Access and egress.*
   1. *Structural ramps.*
      i. Structural ramps that are used solely by employees as a means of access or egress from excavations shall be designed by a competent person. Structural ramps used for access or egress of equipment shall be designed by a competent person qualified in structural design, and shall be constructed in accordance with the design.
      ii. Ramps and runways constructed of two or more structural members shall have the structural members connected together to prevent displacement.
      iii. Structural members used for ramps and runways shall be of uniform thickness.
      iv. Cleats or other appropriate means used to connect runway structural members shall be attached to the bottom of the runway or shall be attached in a manner to prevent tripping.
      v. Structural ramps used in lieu of steps shall be provided with cleats or other surface treatments on the top surface to prevent slipping.
   2. *Means of egress from trench excavations.* A stairway, ladder, ramp, or other safe means of egress shall be located in trench excavations that are 4 feet (1.22 m) or more in depth so as to require no more than 25 feet (7.62 m) of lateral travel for employees.

d. *Exposure to vehicular traffic.* Employees exposed to public vehicular traffic shall be provided with, and shall wear, warning vests or other suitable garments marked with or made of reflectorized or high-visibility material.

e. *Exposure to falling loads.* No employee shall be permitted underneath loads handled by lifting or digging equipment. Employees shall be required to stand away from any vehicle being loaded or unloaded to avoid being struck by any spillage or falling materials. Operators may remain in the cabs of vehicles being loaded or unloaded when the vehicles are equipped, in accordance with §1926.601(b)(6), to provide adequate protection for the operator during loading and unloading operations.

f. *Warning system for mobile equipment.* When mobile equipment is operated adjacent to an excavation, or when such equipment is required to approach the edge of an excavation, and the operator does not have a clear and direct view of the edge of the excavation, a warning system shall be utilized such as barricades, hand or mechanical signals, or stop logs. If possible, the grade should be away from the excavation.

g. *Hazardous atmospheres.*
   1. *Testing and controls.* In addition to the requirements set forth in subparts D and E of this part (29 CFR 1926.50–1926.107) to prevent exposure to harmful levels of atmospheric contaminants and to assure acceptable atmospheric conditions, the following requirements shall apply:
      i. Where oxygen deficiency (atmospheres containing less than 19.5% oxygen) or a hazardous atmosphere exists or could reasonably be expected to exist, such as in excavations in landfill areas or excavations in areas where hazardous substances are stored nearby, the atmospheres in the excavation shall be tested before employees enter excavations greater than 4 feet (1.22 m) in depth.
      ii. Adequate precautions shall be taken to prevent employee exposure to atmospheres containing less than 19.5% oxygen and other hazardous atmospheres.

These precautions include providing proper respiratory protection or ventilation in accordance with subparts D and E of this part respectively.

   iii. Adequate precaution shall be taken such as providing ventilation, to prevent employee exposure to an atmosphere containing a concentration of a flammable gas in excess of 20% of the lower flammable limit of the gas.

   iv. When controls are used that are intended to reduce the level of atmospheric contaminants to acceptable levels, testing shall be conducted as often as necessary to ensure that the atmosphere remains safe.

2. *Emergency rescue equipment.*

   i. Emergency rescue equipment, such as breathing apparatus, a safety harness and line, or a basket stretcher, shall be readily available where hazardous atmospheric conditions exist or may reasonably be expected to develop during work in an excavation. This equipment shall be attended when in use.

   ii. Employees entering bell-bottom pier holes or other similar deep and confined footing excavations, shall wear a harness with a lifeline securely attached to it. The lifeline shall be separate from any line used to handle materials, and shall be individually attended at all times while the employee wearing the lifeline is in the excavation.

h. *Protection from hazards associated with water accumulation.*

1. Employees shall not work in excavations in which there is accumulated water, or in excavations in which water is accumulating, unless adequate precautions have been taken to protect employees against the hazards posed by water accumulation. The precautions necessary to protect employees adequately vary with each situation, but could include special support or shield systems to protect from cave-ins, water removal to control the level of accumulating water, or use of a safety harness and lifeline.

2. If water is controlled or prevented from accumulating by the use of water removal equipment, the water removal equipment and operations shall be monitored by a competent person to ensure proper operation.

3. If excavation work interrupts the natural drainage of surface water (such as streams), diversion ditches, dikes, or other suitable means shall be used to prevent surface water from entering the excavation and to provide adequate drainage of the area adjacent to the excavation. Excavations subject to runoff from heavy rains will require an inspection by a competent person and compliance with paragraphs (h)(1) and (h)(2) of this section.

i. *Stability of adjacent structures.*

1. Where the stability of adjoining buildings, walls, or other structures is endangered by excavation operations, support systems such as shoring, bracing, or underpinning shall be provided to ensure the stability of such structures for the protection of employees.

2. Excavation below the level of the base or footing of any foundation or retaining wall that could be reasonably expected to pose a hazard to employees shall not be permitted except when:

   i. A support system, such as underpinning, is provided to ensure the safety of employees and the stability of the structure; or

   ii. The excavation is in stable rock; or

   iii. A registered professional engineer has approved the determination that the structure is sufficiently removed from the excavation so as to be unaffected by the excavation activity; or

   iv. A registered professional engineer has approved the determination that such excavation work will not pose a hazard to employees.

3. Sidewalks, pavements, and appurtenant structure shall not be undermined unless a support system or another method of protection is provided to protect employees from the possible collapse of such structures.

j. *Protection of employees from loose rock or soil.*

1. Adequate protection shall be provided to protect employees from loose rock or soil that could pose a hazard by falling or rolling from an excavation face. Such protection shall consist of scaling to remove loose material; installation of protective barricades at intervals as necessary on the face to stop and contain falling material; or other means that provide equivalent protection.

2. Employees shall be protected from excavated or other materials or equipment that could pose a hazard by falling or rolling into excavations. Protection shall be pro-

vided by placing and keeping such materials or equipment at least 2 feet (.61 m) from the edge of excavations, or by the use of retaining devices that are sufficient to prevent materials or equipment from falling or rolling into excavations, or by a combination of both if necessary.

k. *Inspections.*

1. Daily inspections of excavations, the adjacent areas, and protective systems shall be made by a competent person for evidence of a situation that could result in possible cave-ins, indications of failure of protective systems, hazardous atmospheres, or other hazardous conditions. An inspection shall be conducted by the competent person prior to the start of work and as needed throughout the shift. Inspections shall also be made after every rainstorm or other hazard increasing occurrence. These inspections are only required when employee exposure can be reasonably anticipated.

2. Where the competent person finds evidence of a situation that could result in a possible cave-in, indications of failure of protective systems, hazardous atmospheres, or other hazardous conditions, exposed employees shall be removed from the hazardous area until the necessary precautions have been taken to ensure their safety.

l. *Fall protection.*

1. Where employees or equipment are required or permitted to cross over excavations, walking ways or bridges with standard guardrails shall be provided.

2. Adquate barrier physical protection shall be provided at all remotely located excavations. All wells, pits, shafts, etc., shall be barricaded or covered. Upon completion of exploration and similar operations, temporary wells, pits, shafts, etc., shall be backfilled.

§1926.652 Requirements for protective systems

a. *Protection of employees in excavations.*

1. Each employee in an excavation shall be protected from cave-ins by an adequate protective system designed in accordance with paragraph (b) or (c) of this section except when:

    i. Excavations are made entirely in stable rock; or

    ii. Excavations are less than 5 feet (1.52m) in depth and examination of the ground by a competent person provides no indication of a potential cave-in.

2. Protective systems shall have the capacity to resist without failure all loads that are intended or could reasonably be expected to be applied or transmitted to the system.

b. *Design of sloping and benching systems.* The slopes and configurations of sloping and benching systems shall be selected and constructed by the employer or his designee and shall be in accordance with the requirements of paragraph (b)(1); or, in the alternative, paragraph (b)(2); or, in the alternative, paragraph (b)(3); or, in the alternative, paragraph (b)(4), as follows:

1. *Option (1)—Allowable configurations and slopes.*

    i. Excavations shall be sloped at an angle not steeper than one and one-half horizontal to one vertical (34° measured from the horizontal), unless the employer uses one of the other options listed below.

    ii. Slopes specified in paragraph (b)(1)(i) of this section, shall be excavated to form configurations that are in accordance with the slopes shown for Type C soil in Appendix B to this subpart.

2. *Option (2)—Determination of slopes and configurations using Appendices A and B.* Maximum allowable slopes, and allowable configurations for sloping and benching systems, shall be determined in accordance with the conditions and requirements set forth in appendices A and B to this subpart.

3. *Option (3)—Designs using other tabulated data.*

    i. Designs of sloping or benching systems shall be selected from and be in accordance with tabulated data, such as tables and charts.

    ii. The tabulated data shall be in written form and shall include all of the following:

        A. Identification of the parameters that affect the selection of a sloping or benching system drawn from such data;

        B. Identification of the limits of use of the data, to include the magnitude and configuration of slopes determined to be safe;

        C. Explanatory information as may be necessary to aid the user in making a correct selection of a protective system from the data.

    iii. At least one copy of the tabulated data which identifies the registered professional engineer who approved the data, shall be maintained at the jobsite during construction of the protective system. After that time the data may be stored off the jobsite, but a copy of the data shall be made available to the Secretary upon request.

4. *Option (4)—Design by a registered professional engineer.*

   i. Sloping and benching systems not utilizing Option (1) or Option (2) or Option (3) under paragraph (b) of this section shall be approved by a registered professional engineer.

   ii. Designs shall be in written form and shall include at least the following:

      A. The magnitude of the slopes that were determined to be safe for the particular project;

      B. The configurations that were determined to be safe for the particular project;

      C. The identity of the registered professional engineer approving the design.

   iii. At least one copy of the design shall be maintained at the jobsite while the slope is being constructed. After that time the design need not be at the jobsite, but a copy shall be made available to the Secretary upon request.

c. *Design of support systems, shield systems, and other protective systems.* Designs of support systems, shield systems, and other protective systems shall be selected and constructed by the employer or his designee and shall be in accordance with the requirements of paragraph (c)(1); or, in the alternative, paragraph (c)(2); or, in the alternative, paragraph (c)(3); or, in the alternative, paragraph (c)(4) as follows:

1. *Option (1)—Designs using appendices A, C and D.* Designs for timber shoring in trenches shall be determined in accordance with the conditions and requirements set forth in appendices A and C to this subpart. Designs for aluminum hydraulic shoring shall be in accordance with paragraph (c)(2) of this section, but if manufacturer's tabulated data cannot be utilized, designs shall be in accordance with appendix D.

2. *Option (2)—Designs Using Manufacturer's Tabulated Data.*

   i. Design of support systems, shield systems, or other protective systems that are drawn from manufacturer's tabulated data shall be in accordance with all specifications, recommendations, and limitations issued or made by the manufacturer.

   ii. Deviation from the specifications, recommendations, and limitations issued or made by the manufacturer shall only be allowed after the manufacturer issues specific written approval.

   iii. Manufacturer's specifications, recommendations, and limitations, and manufacturer's approval to deviate from the specifications, recommendations, and limitations shall be in written form at the jobsite during construction of the protective system. After that time this data may be stored off the jobsite, but a copy shall be made available to the Secretary upon request.

3. *Option (3)—Designs using other tabulated data.*

   i. Designs of support systems, shield systems, or other protective systems shall be selected from and be in accordance with tabulated data, such as tables and charts.

   ii. The tabulated data shall be in written form and include all of the following:

      A. Identification of the parameters that affect the selection of a protective system drawn from such data;

      B. Identification of the limits of use of the data;

      C. Explanatory information as may be necessary to aid the user in making a correct selection of a protective system from the data.

   iii. At least one copy of the tabulated data, which identifies the registered professional engineer who approved the data, shall be maintained at the jobsite during construction of the protective system. After that time the data may be stored off the jobsite, but a copy of the data shall be made available to the Secretary upon request.

4. *Option (4)—Design by a registered professional engineer.*

   i. Support systems, shield systems, and other protective systems not utilizing Option (1), Option (2) or Option (3), above, shall be approved by a registered professional engineer.

   ii. Designs shall be in written form and shall include the following:

      A. A plan indicating the sizes, types, and configurations of the materials to be used in the protective system;

      B. The identity of the registered professional engineer approving the design.

   iii. At least one copy of the design shall be maintained at the jobsite during construction of the protective system. After that time, the design may be stored off the jobsite, but a copy of the design shall be made available to the Secretary upon request.

d. *Materials and equipment.*

1. Materials and equipment used for protective systems shall be free from damage or defects that might impair their proper function.

2. Manufactured materials and equipment used for protective systems shall be used and maintained in a manner that is consistent with the recommendations of the manufacturer, and in a manner that will prevent employee exposure to hazards.

3. When material or equipment that is used for protective systems is damaged, a competent person shall examine the material or equipment and evaluate its suitability for continued use. If the competent person cannot assure the material or equipment is able to support the intended loads or is otherwise suitable for safe use, then such material or equipment shall be removed from service, and shall be evaluated and approved by a registered professional engineer before being returned to service.

e. *Installation and removal of support.*

1. *General.*

   i. Members of support systems shall be securely connected together to prevent sliding, falling, kickouts, or other predictable failure.

   ii. Support systems shall be installed and removed in a manner that protects employees from cave-ins, structural collapses, or from being struck by members of the support system.

   iii. Individual members of support systems shall not be subjected to loads exceeding those which those members were designed to withstand.

   iv. Before temporary removal of individual members begins, additional precautions shall be taken to ensure the safety of employees, such as installing other structural members to carry the loads imposed on the support system.

   v. Removal shall begin at, and progress from, the bottom of the excavation. Members shall be released slowly so as to note any indication of possible failure of the remaining members of the structure or possible cave-in of the sides of the excavation.

   vi. Backfilling shall progress together with the removal of support systems from excavations.

2. *Additional requirements for support systems for trench excavations.*

   i. Excavation of material to a level no greater than 2 feet (.61 m) below the bottom of the members of a support system shall be permitted, but only if the system is designed to resist the forces calculated for the full depth of the trench, and there are no indications while the trench is open of a possible loss of soil from behind or below the bottom of the support system.

   ii. Installation of a support system shall be closely coordinated with the excavation of trenches.

f. *Sloping and benching systems.* Employees shall not be permitted to work on the faces of sloped or benched excavations at levels above other employees except when employees at the lower levels are adequately protected from the hazard of falling, rolling, or sliding material or equipment.

g. *Shield systems.*

1. *General.*

   i. Shield systems shall not be subjected to loads exceeding those which the system was designed to withstand.

   ii. Shields shall be installed in a manner to restrict lateral or other hazardous movement of the shield in the event of the application of sudden lateral loads.

   iii. Employees shall be protected from the hazard of cave-ins when entering or exiting the areas protected by shields.

   iv. Employees shall not be allowed in shields when shields are being installed, removed, or moved vertically.

2. *Additional requirement for shield systems used in trench excavations.* Excavations of earth material to a level not greater than 2 feet (.61 m) below the bottom of a shield shall be permitted, but only if the shield is designed to resist the forces calculated for the full depth of the trench, and there are no indications while the trench is open of a possible loss of soil from behind or below the bottom of the shield.

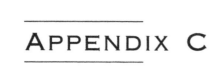

APPENDIX C

Soil Classification

(Adapted from Appendix A to Subpart P—OSHA 29 CFR Ch. XVII)

a. *Scope and application*.
1. *Scope.* This appendix describes a method of classifying soil and rock deposits based on site and environmental conditions, and on the structure and composition of the earth deposits. The appendix contains definitions, sets forth requirements, and describes acceptable visual and manual tests for use in classifying soils.
2. *Application.* This appendix applies when a sloping or benching system is designed in accordance with the requirements set forth in §1926.652(b)(2) as a method of protection for employees from cave-ins. This appendix also applies when timber shoring for excavations is designed as a method of protection from cave-ins in accordance with Appendix C to Subpart P of part 1926, and when aluminum hydraulic shoring is designed in accordance with Appendix D. This appendix also applies if other protective systems are designed and selected for use from data prepared in accordance with the requirements set forth in §1926.652(c), and the use of the data is predicated on the use of the soil classification systen set forth in this appendix.
b. *Definitions.* The definitions and examples given below are based on, in whole or in part, the following: American Society for Testing Materials (ASTM) Standards D653-85 and D2488; The Unified Soils Classification System, The U.S. Department of Agriculture (USDA) Textural Classification Scheme; and The National Bureau of Standards Report BSS-121.
Cemented soil means a soil in which the particles are held together by a chemical agent, such as calcium carbonate, such that a handsize sample cannot be crushed into powder or individual soil particles by finger pressure.
Cohesive soil means clay (fine grained soil), or soil with a high clay content, which has cohesive strength. Cohesive soil does not crumble, can be excavated with vertical sideslopes, and is plastic when moist. Cohesive soil is hard to break up when dry, and exhibits significant cohesion when submerged. Cohesive soils include clayey silt, sandy clay, silty clay, clay, and organic clay.
Dry soil means soil that does not exhibit visible signs of moisture content.
Fissured means a soil material that has a tendency to break along definite planes of fracture with little resistance, or a material that exhibits open cracks, such as tension cracks, in an exposed surface.
Granular soil means gravel, sand, or silt (coarse grained soil), with little or no clay content. Granular soil has no cohesive strength. Some moist granular soils exhibit apparent cohesion. Granular soil cannot be molded when moist and crumbles easily when dry.
Layered system means two or more distinctly different soil or rock types arranged in layers. Micaceous seams or weakened planes in rock or shale are considered layered.
Moist soil means a condition in which a soil looks and feels damp. Moist cohesive soil can easily be shaped into a ball and rolled into small diameter threads before crumbling. Moist granular soil that contains some cohesive material will exhibit signs of

cohesion between particles.

Plastic means a property of a soil which allows the soil to be deformed or molded without cracking or appreciable volume change.

Saturated soil means a soil in which the voids are filled with water. Saturation does not require flow. Saturation, or near saturation, is necessary for the proper use of instruments such as a pocket penetrometer or sheer vane.

Soil classification system means, for the purpose of this subpart, a method of categorizing soil and rock deposits in a hierarchy of Stable Rock, Type A, Type B, and Type C, in decreasing order of stability. The categories are determined based on an analysis of the properties and performance characteristics of the deposits and the environmental conditions of exposure.

Stable rock means natural solid mineral matter that can be excavated with vertical sides and remain intact while exposed.

Submerged soil means soil which is underwater or is free seeping.

Type A means cohesive soils with an unconfined compressive strength of 1.5 ton per square foot (tsf) (144 kPa) or greater. Examples of cohesive soils are: clay, silty clay, sandy clay, clay loam and, in some cases, silty clay loam and sandy clay loam. Cemented soils such as caliche and hardpan are also considered Type A. However, no soil is Type A if:

  i. The soil is fissured; or

  ii. The soil is subject to vibration from heavy traffic, pile driving, or similar effects; or

  iii. The soil has been previously disturbed; or

  iv. The soil is part of a sloped, layered system where the layers dip into the excavation on a slope of four horizontal to one vertical (4H:1V) or greater; or

  v. The material is subject to other factors that would require it to be classified as a less stable material.

§1926.651 General requirements.

Type B means:

  i. Cohesive soil with an unconfined compressive strength greater than 0.5 tsf (48 kPa) but less than 1.5 tsf (144 kPa); or

  ii. Granular cohesionless soils including: angular gravel (similar to crushed rock), silt, silty loam, sandy loam and, in some cases, silty clay loam and sandy clay loam.

  iii. Previously disturbed soils except those which would otherwise be classified as Type C soil.

  iv. Soil that meets the unconfined compressive strength or cementation requirements for Type A, but is fissured or subject to vibration; or

  v. Dry rock that is not stable; or

  vi. Material that is part of a sloped, layered system where the layers dip into the excavation on a slope less than four horizontal to one vertical (4H:1V), but only if the material would otherwise be classified as Type B.

Type C means:

  i. Cohesive soil with an unconfined compressive strength of 0.5 tsf (48 kPa) or less; or

  ii. Granular soils including gravel, sand, and loamy sand; or

  iii. Submerged soil or soil from which water is freely seeping; or

  iv. Submerged rock that is not stable, or

  v. Material in a sloped, layered system where the layers dip into the excavation or a slope of four horizontal to one vertical (4H:1V) or steeper.

Unconfined compressive strength means the load per unit area at which a soil will fail in compression. It can be determined by laboratory testing, or estimated in the field using a pocket penetrometer, by thumb penetration tests, and other methods.

Wet soil means soil that contains significantly more moisture than moist soil, but in such a range of values that cohesive material will slump or begin to flow when vibrated. Granular material that would exhibit cohesive properties when moist will lose those cohesive properties when wet.

c. *Requirements.*

  1. *Classification of soil and rock deposits.* Each soil and rock deposit shall be classified by a competent person as Stable Rock, Type A, Type B, or Type C in accordance with the definitions set forth in paragraph (b) of this appendix.

  2. *Basis of classification.* The classification of the deposits shall be made based on the

results of at least one visual and at least one manual analysis. Such analyses shall be conducted by a competent person using tests described in paragraph (d) below, or in other recognized methods of soil classification and testing such as those adopted by the American Society for Testing Materials, or the U.S. Department of Agriculture Textural Classification Scheme.

3. *Visual and manual analyses.* The visual and manual analyses, such as those noted as being acceptable in paragraph (d) of this appendix, shall be designed and conducted to provide sufficient quantitative and qualitative information as may be necessary to identify properly the properties, factors, and conditions affecting the classification of the deposits.

4. *Layered systems.* In a layered system, the system shall be classified in accordance with its weakest layer. However, each layer may be classified individually where a more stable layer lies under a less stable layer.

5. *Reclassification.* If, after classifying a deposit, the properties, factors, or conditions affecting its classification change in any way, the changes shall be evaluated by a competent person. The deposit shall be reclassified as necessary to reflect the changed circumstances.

d. *Acceptable visual and manual tests.*

1. *Visual tests.* Visual analysis is conducted to determine qualitative information regarding the excavation site in general, the soil adjacent to the excavation, the soil forming the sides of the open excavation, and the soil taken as samples from excavated material.

   i. Observe samples of soil that are excavated and soil in the sides of the excavation. Estimate the range of particle sizes and the relative amounts of the particle sizes. Soil that is primarily composed of fine-grained material is cohesive material. Soil composed primarily of coarse-grained sand or gravel is granular material.

   ii. Observe soil as it is excavated. Soil that remains in clumps when excavated is cohesive. Soil that breaks up easily and does not stay in clumps is granular.

   iii. Observe the side of the opened excavation and the surface area adjacent to the excavation. Crack-like openings such as tension cracks would indicate fissured material. If chunks of soil spall off a vertical side, the soil could be fissured. Small spalls are evidence of moving ground and are indications of potentially hazardous situations.

   iv. Observe the area adjacent to the excavation and the excavation itself for evidence of existing utility and other underground structures, and to identify previously disturbed soil.

   v. Observe the opened side of the excavation to identify layered systems. Examine layered systems to identify if the layers slope toward the excavation. Estimate the degree of slope of the layers.

   vi. Observe the area adjacent to the excavation and the sides of the opened excavation for evidence of surface water, water seeping from the sides of the excavation, or the location of the level of the water table.

   vii. Observe the area adjacent to the excavation and the area within the excavation for sources of vibration that may affect the stability of the excavation face.

2. *Manual tests.* Manual analysis of soil samples is conducted to determine quantitative as well as qualitative properties of soil and to provide more information in order to classify soil properly.

   i. *Plasticity.* Mold a moist or wet sample of soil into a ball and attempt to roll it into threads as thin as ⅛-inch in diameter. Cohesive material can be successfully rolled into threads without crumbling. For example, if at least a 2 inch (50 mm) length of ⅛-inch thread can be held on one end without tearing, the soil is cohesive.

   ii. *Dry strength.* If the soil is dry and crumbles on its own or with moderate pressure into individual grains or fine powder, it is granular (any combination of gravel, sand, or silt). If the soil is dry and falls into clumps which break up into smaller clumps, but the smaller clumps can only be broken up with difficulty, it may be clay in any combination with gravel, sand, or silt. If the dry soil breaks into clumps which do not break up into small clumps and which can only be broken with difficulty, and there is no visual indication the soil is fissured, the soil may be considered unfissured.

   iii. *Thumb penetration.* The thumb penetration test can be used to estimate the unconfined compressive strength of cohesive soils. (This test is based on the thumb penetration test described in American Society for Testing and Materials (ASTM) Standard designation D2488—"Standard Recommended Practice for Description of Soils (Visual—Manual Procedure)." Type A soils with an unconfined compressive strength of 1.5 tsf can be readily indented by the thumb; however, they can be penetrated by the thumb only with very great effort. Type C soils with an unconfined compressive strength of 0.5 tsf can be easily penetrated several inches by the thumb, and can be molded by light finger pressure. This test should be conducted on an undisturbed soil sample, such as a large clump of spoil, as soon as practicable after excavation to keep to a minimum the effects of exposure to drying influences. If the excavation is later exposed to wetting influences (rain, flooding), the classification of the soil must be changed accordingly.

    iv. *Other strength tests.* Estimates of unconfined compressive strength of soils can also be obtained by use of a pocket penetrometer or by using a hand-operated shearvane.

    v. *Dying test.* The basic purpose of the drying test is to differentiate between cohesive material with fissures, unfissured cohesive material, and granular material. The procedure for the drying test involves drying a sample of soil that is approximately 1 inch thick (2.54 cm) and 6 inches (15.24 cm) in diameter until it is thoroughly dry.

        A. If the sample develops cracks as it dries, significant fissures are indicated.

        B. Samples that dry without cracking are to be broken by hand. If considerable force is necessary to break a sample, the soil has significant cohesive material content. The soil can be classified as an unfissured cohesive material and the unconfined compressive strength should be determined.

        C. If a sample breaks easily by hand, it is either a fissured cohesive material or a granular material. To distinguish between the two, pulverize the dried clumps of the sample by hand or by stepping on them. If the clumps do not pulverize easily, the material is cohesive with fissures. If they pulverize easily into very small fragments, the material is granular.

Appendix B to Subpart P—Sloping and Benching

a. *Scope and application.* This appendix contains specifications for sloping and benching when used as methods of protecting employees working in excavations from cave-ins. The requirements of this appendix apply when the design of sloping and benching protective systems is to be performed in accordance with the requirements set forth in §1926.652(b)(2).

b. *Definitions.*

Actual slope means the slope to which an excavation face is excavated.

Distress means that the soil is in a condition where a cave-in is imminent or is likely to occur. Distress is evidenced by such phenomena as the development of fissures in the face of or adjacent to an open excavation; the subsidence of the edge of an excavation; the slumping of material from the face or the bulging or heaving of material from the bottom of an excavation; the spalling of material from the face of an excavation; and ravelling, i.e., small amounts of material such as pebbles or little clumps of material suddenly separating from the face of an excavation and trickling or rolling down into the excavation.

Maximum allowable slope means the steepest incline of an excavation face that is acceptable for the most favorable site conditions as protection against cave-ins, and is expressed as the ratio of horizontal distance to vertical rise (H:V).

Short-term exposure means a period of time less than or equal to 24 hours that an excavation is open.

c. *Requirements.*

    1. *Soil classification.* Soil and rock deposits shall be classified in accordance with Appendix A to Subpart P of part 1926.

    2. *Maximum allowable slope.* The maximum allowable slope for a soil or rock deposit shall be determined from Table C–1 of this appendix.

    3. *Actual slope.*

      i. The actual slope shall not be steeper than the maximum allowable slope.

      ii. The actual slope shall be less steep than the maximum allowable slope, when

Table C-I ▼ MAXIMUM ALLOWABLE SLOPES	
Soil or Rock Type	Maximum Allowable Slopes (H:V) [1] for Excavators Less than 20 Feet Deep [3]
Stable rock	Vertical (90°)
Type A [2]	3/4:1 (53°)
Type B	1:1 (45°)
Type C	$1\frac{1}{2}$:1 (34°)

1. Numbers shown in parentheses next to maximum allowable slopes are angles expressed in degrees from the horizontal. Angles have been rounded off.

2. A short-term maximum allowable slope of $\frac{1}{2}$H:1V (63°) is allowed in excavations in Type A soil that are 12 feet (3.67 m) or less in depth. Short-term maximum allowable slopes for excavations greater than 12 feet (3.67 m) in depth shall be $\frac{3}{4}$H:1V (53°).

3. Sloping or benching for excavations greater than 20 feet deep shall be designed by a registered professional engineer.

there are signs of distress. If that situation occurs, the slope shall be cut back to an actual slope which is at least ½ horizontal to one vertical (½H:1V) less steep than the maximum allowable slope.

iii. When surcharge loads from stored material or equipment, operating equipment, or traffic are present, a competent person shall determine the degree to which the actual slope must be reduced below the maximum allowable slope, and shall assure that such reduction is achieved. Surcharge loads from adjacent structures shall be evaluated in accordance with §1926.651(i).

4. *Configurations.* Configurations of sloping and benching systems shall be in accordance with Figure C–1.

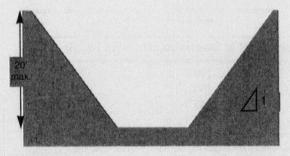

Figure C-1. Simple slope—general.

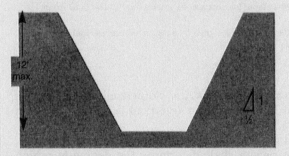

Figure C-2. Simple slope—short term.

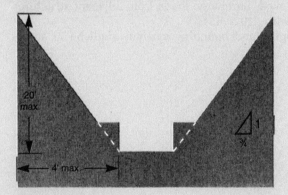

Figure C-3. Simple bench.

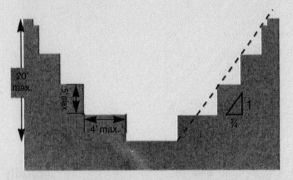

Figure C-4. Unsupported vertically sided lower portion—maximum 12 feet in depth.

SLOPE CONFIGURATION

(All slopes stated below are in the horizontal to vertical ratio)

Excavations Made in Type A Soil.

1. All simple slope excavation 20 feet or less in depth shall have a maximum allowable slope of $\frac{3}{4}$:1.

Exception: Simple slope excavations which are open 24 hours or less (short term) and which are 12 feet or less in depth shall have a maximum allowable slope of $\frac{1}{2}$:1.

2. All benched excavations 20 feet or less in depth shall have a maximum allowable slope of $\frac{3}{4}$ to 1 and maximum bench dimensions as follows:

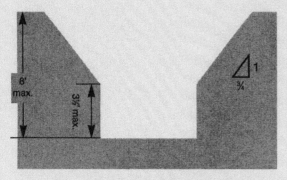

Figure C-5. Unsupported vertically sided lower portion—maximum 8 feet in depth.

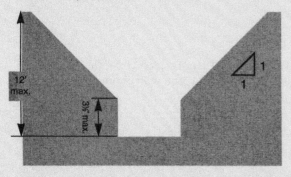

Figure C-6. Unsupported vertically sided lower portion—maximum 12 feet in depth.

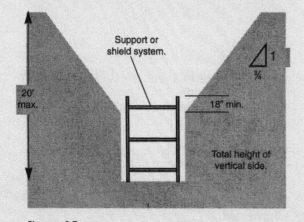

Figure C-7. Supported or shielded vertically sided lower portion.

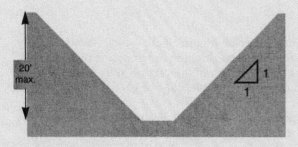

Figure C-8. Simple slope.

3. All excavations of 8 feet or less in depth which have unsupported vertically sided lower portions shall have a maximum vertical side of $3\frac{1}{2}$ feet.

All excavations more than 8 feet but not more than 12 feet in depth which unsupported vertically sided lower portions shall have a maximum allowable slope of 1:1 and a maximum vertical side of $3\frac{1}{2}$ feet.

All excavations 20 feet or less in depth which have vertically sided lower portions that are supported or shielded shall have a maximum allowable slope of $\frac{3}{4}$:1. The support or shield system must extend at least 18 inches above the top of the vertical slide.

4. All other simple slope, compound slope, and vertically sided lower portions excavations shall be in accordance with the other options permitted under §1926.652(b).

Excavations Made in Type B Soil

1. All simple slope excavations 20 feet or less in depth shall have a maximum allowable slope of 1:1.

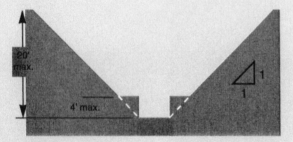

Figure C-9. Single bench.

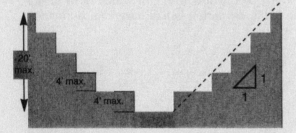

Figure C-10. Multiple bench.

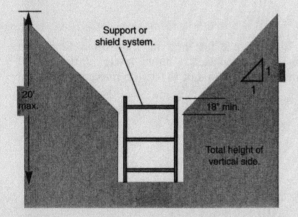

Support or
shield system.

18" min.

Total height of
vertical side.

Figure C-11. Vertically sided lower portion.

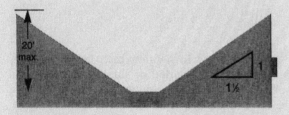

Figure C-12. Simple slope.

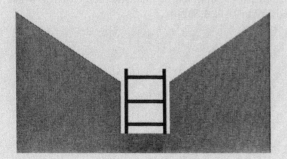

Figure C-13. Vertically sided lower portion.

2. All benched excavations 20 feet or less in depth shall have a maximum allowable slope of 1:1 and maximum bench dimensions as follows:

3. All excavations 20 feet or less in depth which have vertically sided lower portions shall be shielded or supported to a height of at least 18 inches above the top of the vertical side. All such excavations have a maximum allowable slope of 1:1.

4. All other sloped excavations shall be in accordance with the other options permitted in §1926.652(b).

Excavations Made in Type C Soil

1. All simple slope excavations 20 feet or less in depth shall have a maximum allowable slope of $1\frac{1}{2}$:1.

2. All excavations 20 feet or less in depth which have vertically sided lower portions shall be shielded or supported to a height of at least 18 inches above the top of the vertical side. All such excavations have a maximum allowable slope of $1\frac{1}{2}$:1.

3. All other sloped excavations shall be in accordance with the other options permitted in §1926.625(b).

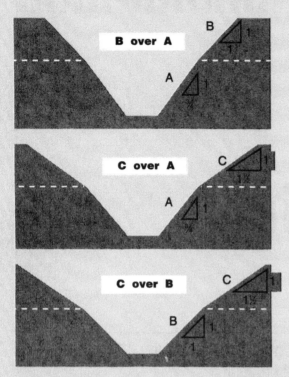

Figure C-14. Layered soils.

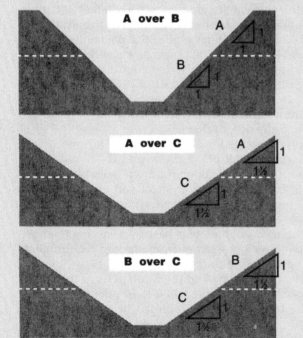

Figure C-15. Layered soils.

Excavations Made in Layered Soil

1. All excavations 20 feet or less in depth made in layered soils shall have a maximum allowable slope for each layer as set forth below.

2. All other sloped excavations shall be in accordance with the other options permitted in §1926.652(b).

Appendix D

Timber Shoring for Trenches

(Adapted from Appendix C to Subpart P—OSHA 29 CFR Ch. XVII)

a. *Scope.* This appendix contains information that can be used if timber shoring is provided as a method of protection from cave-ins in trenches that do not exceed 20 feet (6.1 m) in depth. This appendix must be used when design of timber shoring protective systems is to be performed in accordance with §1926.652(c)(1). Other timber shoring configurations; other systems of support such as hydraulic and pneumatic systems; and other protective systems such as sloping, benching, shielding, and freezing systems must be designed in accordance with the requirements set forth in §1926.652(b) and §1926.652(c).

b. *Soil classification.* In order to use the data presented in this appendix, the soil type or types in which the excavation is made must first be determined using the soil classification method set forth in Appendix A of Subpart P of this part.

c. *Presentation of information.* Information is presented in several forms as follows:

1. Information is presented in tabular form in Tables D–1, D–2, and D–3, and Tables D–4, D–5, and D–6 following paragraph (g) of the appendix. Each table presents the minimum sizes of timber members to use in a shoring system, and each table contains data only for the particular soil type in which the excavation or portion of the excavation is made. The data are arranged to allow the user the flexibility to select from among several acceptable configurations of members based on varying the horizontal spacing of the crossbraces. Stable rock is exempt from shoring requirements and therefore, no data are presented for this condition.

2. Information concerning the basis of the tabular data and the limitations of the data is presented in paragraph (d) of this appendix, and on the tables themselves.

3. Information explaining the use of the tabular data is presented in paragraph (e) of this appendix.

4. Information illustrating the use of the tabular data is presented in paragraph (f) of this appendix.

5. Miscellaneous notations regarding Tables C–1.1 through C–1.3 and Tables C–2.1 through C–2.3 are presented in paragraph (g) of this appendix.

d. *Basis and limitations of the data.*

1. *Dimensions of timber members.*

   i. The sizes of the timber members listed in Tables C–1.1 through C–1.3 are taken from the National Bureau of Standards (NBS) report, "Recommended Technical Provisions for Construction Practice in Shoring and Sloping of Trenches and Excavations." In addition, where NBS did not recommend specific sizes of members, member sizes are based on an analysis of the sizes required for use by existing codes and on empirical practice.

   ii. The required dimensions of the members listed in Tables C–1.1 through C–1.3 refer to actual dimensions and not nominal dimensions of the timber. Employers wanting to use nominal size shoring are directed to Tables C–2.1 through C–2.3, or have this choice under §1926.652(c)(3), and are referred to The Corps of Engineers, The Bureau of Reclamation, or data from other acceptable sources.

2. *Limitation of application.*

   i. It is not intended that the timber shoring specification apply to every situation that may be experienced in the field. These data were developed to apply to the situation that may be experienced in the field. These data were developed to apply to the situations that are most commonly experienced in current trenching practice. Shoring systems for use in situations that are not covered by the data in this appendix must be designed as specified in §1926.652(c)

   ii. When any of the following conditions are present, the members specified in the tables are not considered adequate. Either an alternate timber shoring system must be designed or another type of protective system designed in accordance with §1926.652.

      A. When loads imposed by structures or by stored material adjacent to the trench weigh in excess of the load imposed by a 2-foot soil surcharge. The term "adjacent" as used here means the area within a horizontal distance from the edge of the trench equal to the depth of the trench.

      B. When vertical loads imposed on cross braces exceed a 240-pound gravity load distributed on a 1-foot section of the center of the crossbrace.

      C. When surcharge loads are present from equipment weighing in excess of 20,000 pounds.

      D. When only the lower portion of a trench is shored and the remaining portion of the trench is sloped or benched unless: the sloped portion is sloped at an angle less steep than three horizontal to one vertical; or the members are selected from the tables for use at a depth which is determined from the top of the overall trench, and not from the toe of the sloped portion.

e. *Use of tables.* The members of the shoring system that are to be selected using this information are the cross braces, the uprights, and the wales, where wales are required. Minimum sizes of members are specified for use in different types of soil. There are six tables of information, two for each soil type. The soil type must first be determined in accordance with the soil classification system described in Appendix A to Subpart P of part 1926. Using the appropriate table, the selection of the size and spacing of the members is then made. The selection is based on the depth and width of the trench where the members are to be installed and, in most instances, the selection is also based on the horizontal spacing of the crossbraces. Instances where a choice of horizontal spacing of crossbracing is available, the horizontal spacing of the crossbraces must be chosen by the user before the size of any member can be determined. When the soil type, the width and depth of the trench, and the horizontal spacing of the crossbraces are known, the size and vertical spacing of the crossbraces, the size and vertical spacing of the wales, and the size and horizontal spacing of the uprights can be read from the appropriate table.

f. *Examples to illustrate the use of Tables C–1.1 through C–1.3.*

   1. *Example 1.*

      A trench dug in Type A soil is 13 feet deep and 5 feet wide.

      From Table C–1.1, for acceptable arrangements of timber can be used.

      ### Arrangement #1

      Space 4 × 4 crossbraces at 6 feet hotizontally and 4 feet vertically.
      Wales are not required.
      Space 3 × 8 uprights at 6 feet horizontally. This arrangement is commonly called "skip shoring."

      ### Arrangement #2

      Space 4 × 6 crossbraces at 8 feet hotizontally and 4 feet vertically.
      Space 8 × 8 wales at 4 feet vertically.
      Space 2 × 6 uprights at 4 feet horizontally.

      ### Arrangement #3

      Space 6 × 6 crossbraces at 10 feet hotizontally and 4 feet vertically.
      Space 8 × 10 wales at 4 feet vertically.
      Space 2 × 6 uprights at 5 feet horizontally.

Arrangement #4

Space 6 × 6 crossbraces at 12 feet hotizontally and 4 feet vertically.
Space 10 × 10 wales at 4 feet vertically.
Space 3 × 8 uprights at 6 feet horizontally.

2. *Example 2.*

A trench dug in Type B soil is 13 feet deep and 5 feet wide. From Table C–1.2, three acceptable arrangements of members are listed.

Arrangement #1

Space 6 × 6 crossbraces at 6 feet hotizontally and 5 feet vertically.
Space 8 × 8 wales at 5 feet vertically.
Space 2 × 6 uprights at 2 feet horizontally.

Arrangement #2

Space 6 × 8 crossbraces at 8 feet hotizontally and 5 feet vertically.
Space 10 × 10 wales at 5 feet vertically.
Space 2 × 6 uprights at 2 feet horizontally.

Arrangement #3

Space 8 × 8 crossbraces at 10 feet hotizontally and 5 feet vertically.
Space 10 × 12 wales at 5 feet vertically.
Space 2 × 6 uprights at 2 feet horizontally.

3. *Example 3.*

A trench dug in Type C soil is 13 feet deep and 5 feet wide.
From Table C–1.3, two acceptable arrangements of members can be used.

Arrangement #1

Space 8 × 8 crossbraces at 6 feet hotizontally and 5 feet vertically.
Space 10 × 12 wales at 5 feet vertically.
Position 2 × 6 uprights as closely together as possible.
If water must be retained use special tongue and groove uprights to form tight sheeting.

Arrangement #2

Space 8 × 10 crossbraces at 8 feet hotizontally and 5 feet vertically.
Space 12 × 12 wales at 5 feet vertically.
Position 2 × 6 uprights in a close sheeting configuration unless water pressure must be resisted. Tight sheeting must be used where water must be retained.

4. *Example 4.*

A trench dug in Type C soil is 20 feet deep and 11 feet wide. The size and spacing of members for the section of trench that is over 15 feet in depth is determined using Table C–1.3. Only one arrangement of members is provided.
Space 8 × 10 crossbraces at 6 feet hotizontally and 5 feet vertically.
Space 12 × 12 wales at 5 feet vertically.
Use 3 × 6 tight sheeting.
Use of Tables C–2.1 through C–2.3 would follow the same procedures.

g. *Notes for all tables.*

1. Member sizes at spacings other than indicated are to be determined as specified in §1926.652(c), "Design of Protective Systems."
2. When conditions are saturated or submerged use tight sheeting. Tight sheeting refers to the use of specially-edged timber planks (e.g., tongue and groove) at least 3 inches thick, steel sheet piling, or similar construction that when driven or placed in position provide a tight wall to resist the lateral pressure of water and to prevent the loss of backfill material. Close sheeting refers to the placement of planks side-by-side allowing at little space as possible between them.
3. All spacing indicated is measured center to center.
4. Wales to be installed with greater dimension horizontal.
5. If the vertical distance from the center of the lowest crossbrace to the bottom of the trench exceeds 2 and ½ feet, uprights shall be firmly embedded or a mudsill

shall be used. Where uprights are embedded, the vertical distance from the center of the lowest crossbrace to the bottom of the trench shall not exceed 36 inches. When mudsills are used, the vertical distance shall not exceed 42 inches. Mudsills are wales that are installed at the toe of the trench side.

6. Trench jacks may be used in lieu of or in combination with timber crossbraces.
7. Placement of crossbraces. When the vertical spacing of crossbraces is 4 feet, place the top crossbrace no more than 2 feet below the top of the trench. When the vertical spacing of crossbraces is 5 feet, place the top crossbrace no more than 2 and ½ feet below the top of the trench.

Table D–1 ▨ TIMBER TRENCH SHORING—MINIMUM TIMBER REQUIREMENTS*

Soil Type A $P_a = 25 \times H + 72$ psf (2 ft surcharge)

Depth of Trench (Feet)	Horiz. Spacing (Feet)	Cross Braces — Width of Trench (Feet) Up To 4	Up To 6	Up To 9	Up To 12	Up To 15	Vert. Spacing (Feet)	Wales Size (In)	Wales Vert. Spacing (Feet)	Uprights — Max Allowable Horizontal Spacing (Feet) Close	4	5	6	8
5 to 10	Up to 6	4x4	4x4	4x6	6x6	6x6	4	Not Req'd	—				2x6	
	Up to 8	4x4	4x4	4x6	6x6	6x6	4	Not Req'd	—					2x8
	Up to 10	4x6	4x6	4x6	6x6	6x6	4	8x8	4			2x6		
	Up to 12	4x6	4x6	6x6	6x6	6x6	4	8x8	4				2x6	
10 to 15	Up to 6	4x4	4x4	4x6	6x6	6x6	4	Not Req'd	—				3x8	
	Up to 8	4x6	4x6	6x6	6x6	6x6	4	8x8	4		2x6			
	Up to 10	6x6	6x5	6x6	6x8	6x8	4	8x10	4			2x6		
	Up to 12	6x6	6x6	6x6	6x8	6x8	4	10x10	4				3x8	
15 to 20	Up to 6	6x6	6x6	6x6	6x8	6x8	4	6x8	4	3x6				
	Up to 8	6x6	6x6	6x6	6x8	6x8	4	8x8	4	3x6				
	Up to 10	8x8	8x8	8x8	8x8	8x10	4	8x10	4	3x6				
	Up to 12	8x8	8x8	8x8	8x8	8x10	4	10x10	4	3x6				
Over 20	See Note 1													

*Mixed oak or equivalent with a bending strength not less than 850 psi.

**Manufactured members of equivalent strength may by substituted for wood.

Table D—2 ▌ TIMBER TRENCH SHORING—MINIMUM TIMBER REQUIREMENTS*
Soil Type B $P_a = 45 \times H + 72$ psf (2 ft. surcharge)

Depth of Trench (Feet)	Horiz. Spacing (Feet)	Cross Braces — Width of Trench (Feet)					Vert. Spacing (Feet)	Wales Size (In)	Wales Vert. Spacing (Feet)	Uprights — Maximum Allowable Horizontal Spacing (Feet)				
		Up To 4	Up To 6	Up To 9	Up To 12	Up To 15				Close	2	3		
5 to 10	Up to 6	4x6	4x6	6x6	6x6	6x6	5	6x8	5		2x6	2x6		
	Up to 8	6x6	6x6	6x6	6x8	6x8	5	8x10	5			2x6		
	Up to 10	6x6	6x6	6x6	6x8	6x8	5	10x10	5			2x6		
	See Note 1													
10 to 15	Up to 6	6x6	6x6	6x6	6x8	6x8	5	8x8	5		2x6			
	Up to 8	6x8	6x8	6x8	8x8	8x8	5	10x10	5		2x6			
	Up to 10	8x8	8x8	8x8	8x8	8x10	5	10x12	5		2x6			
	See Note 1													
15 to 20	Up to 6	6x8	6x8	6x8	8x8	8x8	5	8x10	5	3x6				
	Up to 8	8x8	8x8	8x8	8x8	8x10	5	10x12	5	3x6				
	Up to 10	8x10	8x10	8x10	8x10	10x10	5	12x12	5	3x6				
	See Note 1													
Over 20	See Note 1													

*Mixed oak or equivalent with a bending strength not less than 850 psi.

**Manufactured members of equivalent strength may by substituted for wood.

Table D-3 ■ TIMBER TRENCH SHORING—MINIMUM TIMBER REQUIREMENTS*
Soil Type C P_a = 80 x H + 72 psf (2 ft. surcharge)

Depth of Trench (Feet)	Horiz. Spacing (Feet)	Cross Braces					Vert. Spacing (Feet)	Size (In)	Vert. Spacing (Feet)	Uprights				
		Width of Trench (Feet)								Maximum Allowable Horizontal Spacing (Feet) (See Note 2)				
		Up To 4	Up To 6	Up To 9	Up To 12	Up To 15				Close				
5 to 10	Up to 6	6x8	6x8	6x8	8x8	8x8	5	8x10	5	2x6				
	Up to 8	8x8	8x8	8x8	8x8	8x10	5	10x12	5	2x6				
	Up to 10	8x10	8x10	8x10	8x10	8x10	5	12x12	5	2x6				
	See Note 1													
10 to 15	Up to 6	8x8	8x8	8x8	8x8	8x10	5	10x12	5	2x6				
	Up to 8	8x10	8x10	8x10	8x10	10x10	5	12x12	5	2x6				
	See Note 1													
	See Note 1													
15 to 20	Up to 6	8x10	8x10	8x10	8x10	10x10	5	12x12	5	3x6				
	See Note 1													
	See Note 1													
	See Note 1													
Over 20	See Note 1													

*Mixed oak or equivalent with a bending strength not less than 850 psi.

**Manufactured members of equivalent strength may be substituted for wood.

Table D–4 ◢ TIMBER TRENCH SHORING—MINIMUM TIMBER REQUIREMENTS*
Soil Type A $P_a = 25 \times H + 72$ psf (2 ft. surcharge)

Depth of Trench (Feet)	Horiz. Spacing (Feet)	Cross Braces — Width of Trench (Feet)					Vert. Spacing (Feet)	Wales Size (In)	Wales Vert. Spacing (Feet)	Uprights — Maximum Allowable Horizontal Spacing (Feet)				
		Up To 4	Up To 6	Up To 9	Up To 12	Up To 15				Close	4	5	6	8
5 to 10	Up to 6	4x4	4x4	4x4	4x4	4x6	4	Not Req'd	Not Req'd				4x6	
	Up to 8	4x4	4x4	4x4	4x6	4x6	4	Not Req'd	Not Req'd					4x8
	Up to 10	4x6	4x6	4x6	6x6	6x6	4	8x8	4			4x6		
	Up to 12	4x6	4x6	4x6	6x6	6x6	4	8x8	4				4x6	
10 to 15	Up to 6	4x4	4x4	4x4	6x6	6x6	4	Not Req'd	Not Req'd				4x10	
	Up to 8	4x6	4x6	4x6	6x6	6x6	4	6x8	4		4x6			
	Up to 10	6x6	6x6	6x6	6x8	6x6	4	8x8	4			4x8		
	Up to 12	6x6	6x6	6x6	6x6	6x6	4	8x10	4		4x6		4x10	
15 to 20	Up to 6	6x6	6x6	6x6	6x6	6x6	4	6x8	4	3x6				
	Up to 8	6x6	6x6	6x6	6x6	6x6	4	8x8	4	3x6	4x12			
	Up to 10	6x6	6x6	6x6	6x6	6x8	4	8x10	4	3x6				
	Up to 12	6x6	6x6	6x6	6x8	6x8	4	8x12	4	3x6	4x12			
Over 20	See Note 1													

*Douglas fir or equivalent with a bending strength not less than 1500 psi.

**Manufactured members of equivalent strength may be substituted for wood.

Table D–5 ▮ TIMBER TRENCH SHORING — MINIMUM TIMBER REQUIREMENTS*

Soil Type B $P_a = 45 \times H + 72$ psf (2 ft. surcharge)

Depth of Trench (Feet)	Horiz. Spacing (Feet)	Cross Braces — Width of Trench (Feet)					Vert. Spacing (Feet)	Wales Size (In)	Wales Vert. Spacing (Feet)	Uprights — Maximum Allowable Horizontal Spacing (Feet)				
		Up To 4	Up To 6	Up To 9	Up To 12	Up To 15				Close	2	3	4	6
5 to 10	Up to 6	4x6	4x6	4x6	6x6	6x6	5	6x8	5			3x12 4x8		4x12
	Up to 8	4x6	4x6	6x6	6x6	6x6	5	8x8	5		3x8		4x8	
	Up to 10	4x6	4x6	6x6	6x6	6x8	5	8x10	5			4x8		
	See Note 1													
10 to 15	Up to 6	6x6	6x6	6x6	6x8	6x8	5	8x8	5	3x6	4x10			
	Up to 8	6x8	6x8	6x8	8x8	8x8	5	10x10	5	3x6	4x10			
	Up to 10	6x8	8x8	6x8	8x8	8x8	5	10x12	5	3x6	4x10			
	See Note 1													
15 to 20	Up to 6	6x8	6x8	6x8	6x8	8x8	5	8x10	5	4x6				
	Up to 8	6x8	6x8	6x8	8x8	8x8	5	10x12	5	4x6				
	Up to 10	8x8	8x8	6x8	8x8	8x8	5	12x12	5	4x6				
	See Note 1													
Over 20	See Note 1													

*Douglas fir or equivalent with a bending strength not less than 1500 psi.

**Manufactured members of equivalent strength may be substituted for wood.

Table D-6 TIMBER TRENCH SHORING—MINIMUM TIMBER REQUIREMENTS*

Soil Type C $P_a = 80 \times H + 72$ psf (2 ft. surcharge)

Depth of Trench (Feet)	Horiz. Spacing (Feet)	Size (Actual) and Spacing of Members**													
		Cross Braces						Wales		Uprights					
		Width of Trench (Feet)					Vert. Spacing (Feet)	Size (In)	Vert. Spacing (Feet)	Maximum Allowable Horizontal Spacing (Feet)					
		Up To 4	Up To 6	Up To 9	Up To 12	Up To 15				Close					
5 to 10	Up to 6	6x6	6x6	6x6	6x6	8x8	5	8x8	5	3x6					
	Up to 8	6x6	6x6	6x6	8x8	8x8	5	10x10	5	3x6					
	Up to 10	6x6	6x6	8x8	8x8	8x8	5	10x12	5	3x6					
	See Note 1														
10 to 15	Up to 6	6x8	6x8	6x8	8x8	8x8	5	10x10	5	4x6					
	Up to 8	8x8	8x8	8x8	8x8	8x8	5	12x12	5	4x6					
	See Note 1														
	See Note 1														
15 to 20	Up to 6	8x8	8x8	8x8	8x10	8x10	5	10x12	5	4x6					
	See Note 1														
	See Note 1														
	See Note 1														
Over 20	See Note 1														

*Douglas fir or equivalent with a bending strength not less than 1500 psi.

**Manufactured members of equivalent strength may be substituted for wood.

Glossary

Angle of repose. The greatest angle above the horizontal plane at which loose material (such as soil) will lie without sliding.

Asphyxiant. A gas capable of causing death from oxygen deficiency.

Atmospheric monitor. A device used to analyze oxygen content, hydrocarbons, and toxic gases.

Backboard. A rigid, full-body immobilization device generally 6 feet long by 18 to 24 inches wide and made of wood; often called a long spine board.

Backfill. The refilling of a trench; or, as a noun, the material used to refill a trench.

Backhoe. An excavating machine that is equipped with an articulating boom and a bucket. May have crawler tracks or rubber tires.

Basket stretcher. A basket-like, formed wire or plastic patient-carrying device designed to afford maximum protection for a person who must be moved over rough terrain.

Batter boards. A series of horizontal boards spanning a trench, used by the contractor to set the line and grade of a pipe.

Bedding. Sand or fine stone that is placed in the bottom of a trench as the foundation for a pipe.

Bedding stone. Small rocks spread over the floor of a trench as a foundation for sewer pipes and other utility lines.

Bisect. To cross or intersect.

Blockade. A barrier placed to halt the flow of vehicle traffic.

Boxed end of the shore. The end of a timber shore that is held in place against the sheeting with scabs.

Bulldozer. A crawler-equipped machine with a large horizontal blade designed for land clearing, material moving, etc.

Burr. A rough protrusion from the face of a metal part.

Cardiac arrest. A sudden cessation of heart action followed by the loss of arterial blood pressure.

Cardiopulmonary resuscitation. The combination of chest compressions and ventilations provided by rescuers in an effort to restore spontaneous breathing and heart action in a person who has suffered cardiac arrest.

Carotid pulse. The rhythmic expansion of the large arteries on both sides of the neck; easily felt with the fingertips.

Catch basin. A precast or built in concrete box that is generally used in storm sewer construction.

Cathead. A shore running between walers, with a 6-inch longer plank nailed to the top.

Cave-in. The collapse of unsupported trench walls.

Cerebrospinal fluid. The clear, watery fluid that helps protect the brain and spinal cord.

Cervical collar. A semi-rigid adjustable collar that partially stabilizes the neck after an injury.

Check. A lengthwise separation of wood fibers, usually extending across the annular rings. Checks commonly result from stresses set up in wood during the seasoning process.

Choke. To pass the end of a wire rope sling through the eye of the other end and pull it until it fastens securely around the object that is to be lifted.

Choker. Another term for wire rope sling.

Clamp stick. A nonconducting lineman's tool essential to the safe movement of energized electric wires.

Closed wound. An injury in which the skin is not broken.

Cohesive. Holding together firmly.

Command post. A place in which the officer in charge of an emergency situation can meet with other emergency service and community resource personnel. May be in a vehicle or a nearby building. Should have communication links with the dispatch center and other services.

Command post kit. A briefcase, trunk, or other container filled with maps, standard operating procedures, directories, community resource lists, inventories, and other items that will help an officer best utilize emergency service forces at the scene of a large-scale incident.

Community resource. A firm or other organization that can provide personnel, equipment, and machines at the time of an emergency.

Compact soil. Soil that is hard and stable in appearance. Compact soil can be readily indented by the thumb but penetrated only with great difficulty.

Confined area. Any space that lacks ventilation; usually the space is larger than the point of entry.

Contusion. A bruise.

Crepitation. The crackling sound that is produced when broken bone ends rub together.

Cribbing. Short pieces of lumber used to support and stabilize an object.

Cul-de-sac. A dead-end street, usually provided with a turnaround at the end.

Cut sheet. A job foreman's daily plan. Shows depth and grades for pipe.

D

Damage. With regard to lumber: injuries such as gouges, splits, and punctures.

Danger zone. The area surrounding an accident site. The size of a danger zone is proportional to the severity of on-the-scene hazards.

Decay. The decomposition of wood substances as a result of fungi.

Deep-well system. A means for dewatering the ground around a trench. In a line parallel to the trench, pipe casings with screens are inserted into the ground to a level below that of the trench floor. Electric submersible pumps lowered into the casings continually dewater the work area. The water is collected in a header and discharged at a point distant from the site.

Detour. A plan or procedure for routing traffic away from the scene of an accident.

Dewatering. Removing water from the work area.

Diaphragm pump. A positive displacement pump that has a diaphragm instead of a piston; an excellent device for moving water in which foreign matter is suspended.

Dilated pupils. Widened pupils of the eyes (as opposed to pupils that are narrowed, or constricted).

Disrupted utilities. Broken water mains, gas mains, service lines, electrical conduits, etc.

Disturbed soil. Ground that has been previously excavated.

Double-head nail. A nail that is provided with a flange close to the head. The flange prevents the nail from being driven all the way. Removal is easy because the head remains exposed.

Downed wires. Electric transmission lines brought down from utility poles by accident.

Driving home pipe. Connecting together pieces of slip-joint pipe.

E

Engineer's hubs. Stakes placed on a utility construction job site by a layout crew.

Euphoria. A feeling of well-being or elation.

Evisceration. Disembowelment; protrusion of the organs through an opening in the abdomen.

Excavation. An opening in the ground that results from a digging effort.

Exposed utilities. Gas mains, water mains, electrical conduits, etc., that are exposed but unbroken during a trench-digging operation.

Extrication collar. A cervical collar with high sides, providing additional protection for the cervical spine.

Eye of the sling. A loop fashioned into the end of a wire rope.

F

Fissure. A narrow opening in the ground; a crack of some length and considerable depth.

Flag stake. A piece of lath with a colored ribbon attached to mark the location of an engineer's hub. Symbols on the stakes tell the contractor where and how deep he should dig.

Flotation. In this case, the distribution of weights and forces over an area of unstable ground.

Freestanding time. The period of time during which trench walls remain unsupported after excavation.

Front-end loader. A rubber tire or crawler-equipped machine with a movable bucket at one end.

Frost line. The depth to which frost penetrates the soil.

G

Gas main. Generally a large-diameter pipeline that carries natural gas under the streets.

Gas service line. A small-diameter pipe that connects the consumer with the gas main under the street.

Grade crossing. A railroad crossing at highway level.

Grade pole. A wood or fiberglass pole that is either cut to a certain length or provided with markings. It is used by workmen when they are setting pipes on grade.

Grease can and brush. A can of lubricant that is helpful for joining slip-joint pipe and the brush with which the lubricant is applied.

Ground cover. A tarpaulin that is placed on the ground for an equipment layout.

Ground pads. Full sheets of $\frac{5}{8}$- or $\frac{3}{4}$-inch plywood placed next to the trench lip. Ground pads distribute weight and forces over their surface area and thus minimize the possibility of rescuers creating a secondary cave-in.

H

Hauling line. A length of rope used to hoist or lower an object.

Haul Safe®. A prerigged lifting and lowering device.

Header. A large-diameter pipe with inlets for suction hoses and a connection for the suction side of a pump.

Hydrostatic pressure. The force generated by a liquid.

Hyperactivity. Excessive activity.

J

Jaw-lift method. A technique for opening the airway by displacing the tongue. The rescuer hooks the jaw of the nonbreathing person between his thumb and forefinger and gently lifts.

Jaw-thrust method. A technique for opening the airway of a nonbreathing person. A forward displacement of the lower jaw by the rescuer causes the tongue to move away from the air passage.

K

Kiln-dried (lumber). Lumber that is artificially dried in an ovenlike structure.

Knot. A hard, irregular lump formed at the point where a branch grows out of the trunk of a tree.

L

Lackluster pupils. Pupils that are dull, lacking the radiance usually associated with the eye.

Landfill. A collection point for trash and garbage. In a sanitary landfill the waste is buried between layers of earth.

Lane control. A procedure for maintaining traffic flow around an accident site by funneling vehicles into fewer lanes.

Language bank. A community resource from which an interpreter can be obtained; usually run by a hospital or a governmental agency.

Laser blower. A motor-driven fan (usually 12 V) used by contractors to purge a pipe of stale air when a laser instrument is being used.

Laser target. A square or triangular plastic device used in conjunction with a laser instrument to set the line and grade of pipe.

Lineman's gloves. A set of nonconducting gum rubber gloves and protective leather shells used when it is necessary to work with a downed wire.

Loam. A combination of sand and clay.

Lower explosive limit. In a range of percentages, the point at which a mixture of flammable gas and air will not ignite because there is an insufficient concentration of the gas.

M

Manhole. An accessway to sewer pipes; an opening used for maintenance and inspection.

Manifold. A pipe fitting with several inlets and/or outlets.

Mechanical strut. An adjustable support. When it is made up into a solid support, it resists forces exerted in the direction of its length.

Mechanism of entrapment. Any object that confines (or traps) an accident victim.

Methane gas. The chief component of natural gas; colorless, odorless, and flammable.

Mine drift. A nearly horizontal mine passageway.

Mobile crane. A crane that is provided with rubber tires for over-the-highway travel.

N

Neck lift–head tilt maneuver. Still another technique for opening the airway. The rescuer places one hand under the person's neck and lifts while he presses on the person's forehead with his other hand.

O

Occlusive material. A nonporous, nonabsorbent

material (such as plastic wrap) that is used to seal an open wound and protect it from air.

Offset. The distance (in feet) perpendicular from an engineer's hub to the pipeline.

One-call system. A service from which contractors, emergency service personnel, and others can obtain information on the location of underground utilities in any area.

Open abdominal wound. An injury in which the abdominal wall has been penetrated.

Open wound. An injury in which the skin is broken and underlying tissues are exposed.

Operating radius (of a crane). The horizontal distance from the centerline of rotation (the center pin of the cab) to a vertical line through the center of gravity of the load.

OSHA. The Occupational Safety and Health Administration, a division of the U.S. Department of Labor.

P

Packaged patient. An injured person who, with wounds dressed and bandaged and fractures immobilized, has been secured to a patient-carrying device.

Pallets. Portable platforms of wood or metal used for the storage and movement of materials and packages.

Panels. Multilayered sheets of wood, usually 4 feet by 8 feet by various thicknesses, used to support the walls of a trench.

Parallel trench. A previously excavated and backfilled trench close to and paralleling the trench being dug.

Parking area. A street or parking area where vehicles not needed in the rescue operation may be safely parked.

Perimeter. In this case, a real or imaginary line established around the accident site to direct the movement of spectators.

Pipe. A conduit for fluids, gases, and finely divided solid materials.

Pipe string. Lengths of pipe laid parallel to the trench lip in preparation for being joined and buried.

Pneumatic shoring. Trench shores or jacks with movable parts that are operated by the action of a compressed gas.

Primary assessment. The initial determination of what has happened in an accident situation; the "size-up."

Profile. A job blueprint that shows sectional elevation.

PVC pipe. A lightweight pipe made of polyvinylchloride.

R

Reeves Sleeve®. A stretcher-like device that can be used for wrapping a victim or as an immobilization device.

Replacement sewer line. A new pipeline installed next to an existing line for the purpose of taking over the original line's function.

Rescue area. Generally the area 50 feet in all directions from the accident site.

Right of way. A strip of land temporarily granted to the contractor so that he can perform his work.

Running soil. Loose, freely flowing soil such as sugar sand.

S

Safing. Making a portion of a trench safe by the installation of sheeting and shoring.

Sanitary sewer. A buried pipeline that carries sewage.

Saturated soil. Soil that contains an unusually high quantity of water. Easily identified because of seeping.

Scab. A short piece of lumber—generally cut from 2- by 4-inch stock—that is nailed to an upright to prevent the shifting of a shore.

Screw jack. A trench shore or jack with interchangeable threaded parts. The threading allows the jack to be lengthened or shortened.

Secondary assessment. A study to see whether on-the-scene capabilities are sufficient to cope with an emergency situation.

Secondary cave-in. A collapse of another portion of a trench wall after the initial accident.

Select fill. Soil that is specially chosen to replace that which has been excavated.

Self-dumping valve. A spring-loaded valve that is part of a pneumatic shoring system. When the valve handle is depressed, the system is pressurized. When the valve handle is released, pressure is released.

Shake. A separation along the grain of lumber.

Shackle. A U-shaped, round piece of steel that is provided with a pin or a threaded bolt. Used to join rigging devices.

Shear. In this case, force-caused stress that results in the sliding of a section of trench wall from the main body of earth.

Sheeting. Generally speaking, wood planks and wood panels that support trench walls when held in place with shoring.

Shorform®. A laminated panel used for sheeting trench walls.

Shoring. The general term used for lengths of timber, screw jacks, pneumatic jacks, and other devices that can be used to hold sheeting against trench walls. Individual supports are called shores, crossbraces, and struts.

Shotgun. Another term for a clamp stick, so named because of the slide action of the wire grip.

Signalman. A person who gives or relays commands to a heavy equipment operator.

Skip-shoring. The procedure for supporting trench walls with uprights and shores at spaced intervals.

Sliding choker. A steel hook provided on a wire rope sling. The hook enables the sling to adjust for loads of various sizes and shapes.

Slope of grain. In lumber, the angle formed between the direction of the fibers and the long axis of the piece; usually expressed as a ratio of rise to run, for example, 1:20.

Slough-in. The collapse of a portion of trench wall in such a fashion that an overhang remains.

Snatch block. A wood- or steel-shell single pulley block that can be opened on one side to accept a rope or cable.

Soil typing. Determining properties of soil such as strength, in-place unit weight, compressibility, and permeability.

Solid sheeting. The procedure for supporting trench walls with sections of sheeting butted together. Also referred to as "closed sheeting."

SOP. Standard operating procedure.

Split. With regard to lumber, a separation of the wood parallel to the fiber direction. Splits result from the tearing apart of wood cells.

Spoil pile. The heap of material excavated from a trench.

Spontaneous breathing. Involuntary, instinctive breathing; breathing that occurs without outside influence.

Spot-bracing. Another term for "skip-shoring."

Spot dewatering. The technique of drawing water from localized portions of the ground around a trench.

Staging area. A gathering point; in this case, for emergency service and support apparatus, equipment, and personnel.

Staging area for essential vehicles. A street or parking area where ambulances, rescue vehicles, and fire apparatus that are essential to the rescue effort are parked.

Storm sewer. A buried pipeline that carries surface water (such as rain water).

Story pole. See *"Grade pole."*

String lines. Strings placed on one side of and parallel to the trench. Used to determine grade.

Strongback. See *"Upright."*

Sucking chest wound. An opening in the chest wall and underlying lung through which air moves in and out with each respiration.

Sump. A pit dug at a low point in a trench floor; it serves to keep the screened end of a suction hose below the water level.

Supplemental sheeting and shoring. Additional sheeting and shoring installed as the level of the trench floor is lowered during digging operations.

Supply point. An area close to the accident site where tools and appliances vital to the rescue effort are stockpiled.

Surcharge. Additional weight in the trench area.

System 99®. A prerigged lifting and lowering device.

T

Tag lines. Handheld lengths of rope—usually $\frac{1}{2}$ inch in diameter—used to steady or move an object that is being hoisted or lowered.

Tension cracks. Cracks in the ground adjacent to the trench. Tension cracks indicate that the ground has shifted; they should be considered warning signs.

Tight sheeting. Tongue-and-grooved timber planks.

Trash pump. A centrifugal or diaphragm pump designed to move water that contains mud, stones, and other debris.

Trench. A temporary excavation that is deeper than it is wide and no wider than 15 feet at the bottom.

Trench box. A steel, fiberglass, or aluminum structure that is placed in a trench to protect workmen from the collapse of the trench walls, and which can be moved along as work progresses.

Trench lip. The edge of a trench.

Tripping hazards. Debris, tools, equipment, and anything else that may cause a person to stumble at a construction site.

U

Unbroken utilities. Water mains, gas mains, electrical conduits, and pipelines that remain intact (although they may be exposed) during a trenching operation.

Underground utilities. Conduits carrying water, gas, electric transmission lines, sewage, etc.

Upper explosive limit. In a range of percentages, the point at which a mixture of flammable gas and air will not ignite because there is not sufficient oxygen.

Uprights. Generally speaking, planks that are held in place against sections of sheeting with shores. Uprights add strength to the shoring system. They distribute forces exerted by trench walls and counterforces exerted by shores over wider areas of the sheeting.

V

Ventilating the trench. Using a powered fan to replace stale or contaminated air in a trench with fresh air.

Virgin soil. Ground that has never been excavated.

W

Wales. Braces that are placed horizontally against sheeting. Wales transmit loading from the sheeting to shores. Also called "walers" and "stringers."

Wall. The side of a trench from the lip to the floor. Also called the "face."

Wane. An edge or corner defect in lumber characterized by the presence of bark or the lack of wood.

Warp. A twist or curve in lumber that was originally straight.

Water main. Generally a large-diameter water-carrying pipeline that is laid under the street.

Water service line. A small-diameter pipe that connects the consumer to the water main.

Water table. The upper limit of a portion of the ground that is wholly saturated with water from underground sources. May be very near the surface or deep in the ground.

Wedged end of the shore. The end of a timber shore opposite the boxed end. It is between this end and the uprights that wedges are driven to make the structure rigid.

Weighted throwing line. One hundred feet of a non-conductive, synthetic-fiber rope used for moving a downed wire when a clamp stick is not available. Steel rings or weighted wood blocks on the ends of the rope aid in achieving distance when the rope is thrown.

Well casing. A large-diameter pipe (12 inches) that is used in deep-well systems.

Well-point system. A series of pipes driven into the ground around a trench for the purpose of dewatering the work area. Water is drawn through the pipes, into a header, and finally into the suction side of a pump.

Whip hose. In a pneumatic shoring system, the length of hose that carries air from the self-dumping valve to the quick-disconnect coupling.

Wire rope. An extremely strong rope made of strands of wire.

Wire rope sling. A lifting device that is made of wire rope. An eye is provided at both ends.

Wire span. The distance between utility poles.

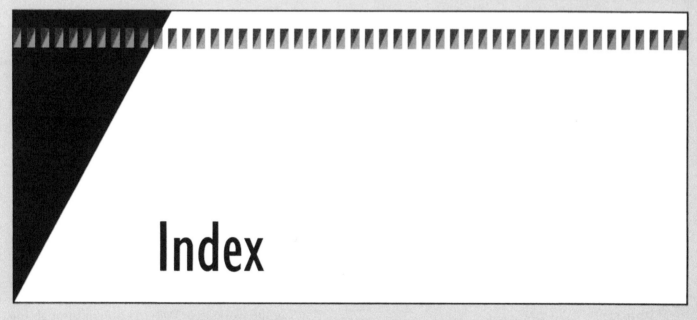

Index

Note: Page numbers followed by "f" designate figures.

About the Author

A resident of Kure Beach, North Carolina, Jim Gargan serves as the president of Rescue Training Consultants.

Mr. Gargan has worked for nearly 50 years in the emergency services field. Having spent all of his active firefighting days with the Prospect Park Fire Department (Pennsylvania), he has served as firefighter, truck captain, rescue captain, battalion chief, deputy chief, and chief of the department before his retirement in 1973.

In 1960, he became a Pennsylvania State Fire School instructor. Teaching at the Lewistown State Fire School, he was senior instructor of the Annual Basic Firefighting Course. From 1961 until 1963, Mr. Gargan was the director of the Delaware County Fire School and was active for many years teaching fire and rescue skills throughout Eastern Pennsylvania. In 1964, the United Clubmen of Delaware County (Pennsylvania) named him Fireman of the Year for outstanding service.

Concurrently with his emergency services career, Mr. Gargan has been closely associated with the heavy construction industry, first as a construction equipment operator and member of the International Union of Operating Engineers, and later as a salesman of heavy construction machinery. He was co-owner of J & B Equipment Company of New Castle, Delaware. Jim Gargan is also the inventor and codeveloper of the Jimmi-Jak® Rescue Tool.

Mr. Gargan is a member of the International Association of Fire Chiefs, the Eastern Association of Fire Chiefs, and the Delaware County (Pennsylvania) Firemen's Association. He also serves on the Advisory Council to the Urban Search and Rescue Task Force of the Congressional Fire Services Caucus in Washington, D.C. Mr. Gargan serves on the Allegheny County (Pennsylvania) Emergency Response Delta Team as a consultant and rigger/specialist. He has appeared in many national seminars and training programs and has written numerous articles for emergency service magazines.

Jim Gargan is the author of *Trench Rescue* and *BTLS Access*. He is the co-author of the second edition of *Vehicle Rescue*, and the *Action Guide for Emergency Service Personnel*.

Printed and bound by CPI Group (UK) Ltd, Croydon, CR0 4YY

03/10/2024

01040349-0020